Early

Learning C   r

Therapy: An ....

"*Learning Cognitive-Behavior Therapy* is an excellent introduction to the nuts and bolts of doing cognitive-behavior therapy. Clear, practical and detailed step-by-step guidelines—accompanied by worksheets and checklists—provide the clinician with the necessary tools to implement effective and powerful interventions. This guide will prove invaluable to those who are learning cognitive-behavior therapy for the first time. The authors are leading authorities in the application of cognitive-behavior therapy and provide the reader with the benefit of their many years of experience."

Robert L. Leahy, Ph.D., President, International Association for Cognitive Psychotherapy; President-Elect, Academy of Cognitive Therapy; Associate Editor, Journal of Cognitive Psychotherapy: An International Quarterly; Professor, Department of Psychiatry, Weill-Cornell University Medical College, New York Hospital; Director, American Institute for Cognitive Therapy

"This is a superior textbook of cognitive-behavior therapy. It will provide psychiatric educators with an ideal tool to help assure that their residents will graduate with competence in CBT. Unlike many cognitive therapy textbooks, this work concentrates on behavioral techniques as well as on more cognitive methods, so that it is useful for a wide range of disorders. The chapter on managing noncompliance with treatment (including with medications) is brilliant and will be useful across virtually all clinical situations. This book is highly recommended and represents a real step forward in psychotherapy training."

Robert M. Goisman, M.D., Associate Professor of Psychiatry, Harvard Medical School; and Director, Medical Student Education, Massachusetts Mental Health Center

Learning Cognitive-Behavior Therapy

An Illustrated Guide

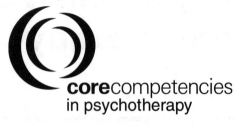

corecompetencies
in psychotherapy

Glen O. Gabbard, M.D., Series Editor

Learning Cognitive-Behavior Therapy

An Illustrated Guide

Jesse H. Wright, M.D., Ph.D.
Professor and Chief of Adult Psychiatry, University of
Louisville School of Medicine, Louisville, Kentucky

Monica R. Basco, Ph.D.
Clinical Associate Professor, Department of Psychiatry,
Division of Psychology, University of Texas Southwestern at
Dallas, Dallas, Texas

Michael E. Thase, M.D.
Professor and Chief of Adult Academic Psychiatry,
University of Pittsburgh Medical Center, Pittsburgh,
Pennsylvania

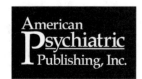

American Psychiatric Publishing, Inc.

Washington, DC
London, England

Manufactured in the United States of America on acid-free paper
09   08   07   06   5   4   3   2
First Edition

Typeset in Adobe's Berling Roman and Frutiger.

American Psychiatric Publishing, Inc.
1000 Wilson Boulevard
Arlington, VA 22209-3901
www.appi.org

Library of Congress Cataloging-in-Publication Data
Learning cognitive-behavior therapy : an illustrated guide / edited by Jesse H. Wright, Monica R. Basco, Michael E. Thase.—1st ed.
    p. ; cm.
    Includes bibliographical references and index.
    ISBN 1-58562-153-6 (pbk. : alk. paper)
    1. Cognitive therapy.
    [DNLM: 1. Cognitive Therapy. WM 425.5.C6 L438 2005] I. Wright, Jesse H.
II. Basco, Monica Ramirez. III. Thase, Michael E.

    RC489.C63L433 2005
    616.89'142—dc22

                                                                    2005014185

British Library Cataloguing in Publication Data
A CIP record is available from the British Library.

Contents

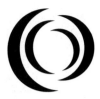

Preface

The influence and reach of cognitive-behavior therapy (CBT) have been growing steadily since this treatment method was introduced in the 1950s. A large number of controlled studies have demonstrated that CBT is an effective treatment for depression, anxiety disorders, and a variety of other conditions. In addition, recent work has shown that CBT adds to the effect of medication in the treatment of persons with severe psychiatric disorders such as refractory depression, bipolar disorder, and schizophrenia. These findings—coupled with the advantages of using a treatment that is focused, pragmatic, and highly collaborative—have fueled interest in learning how to perform CBT.

The inclusion of CBT in the group of therapies for which psychiatry residents must demonstrate competence has added further impetus to the movement to provide effective training in cognitive-behavioral methods. When the principal author of this book (J.H.W.) started to teach CBT to residents, graduate students, and practicing clinicians in the early 1980s, this approach was often viewed as a secondary or specialized therapy. Today, CBT is widely recognized as one of the central organizing theories and methods for the treatment of psychiatric disorders. Courses in CBT are standard offerings in psychiatry residency programs, in psychology graduate training, and in the education of other mental health professionals. Continuing medical education programs for practicing clinicians are offered widely at meetings of the American Psychiatric Association, the American Psychological Association, and many other organizations.

Our goals in writing this book have been to provide an easy-to-use guide to learning the essential skills of CBT and to assist readers in achieving competence in this treatment method. We begin by tracing the origins of the CBT model and giving an overview of core theories and techniques. Next we describe the therapeutic relationship in CBT, explain how to conceptualize a case with the CBT model, and detail effective ways to structure sessions. If you understand these basic features of CBT, you should have a solid platform for learning the specific procedures for changing cognitions and behaviors that are described in the middle chapters of the book (e.g., methods for modifying automatic thoughts; behavioral strategies for treating low energy, lack of interest, and avoidance; and interventions for revising maladaptive core beliefs). The last three chapters of *Learning Cognitive-Behavior Therapy: An Illustrated Guide* are devoted to helping you develop advanced skills such as overcoming obstacles to treatment, treating diverse conditions, and continuing to build knowledge and experience in CBT.

We've found that the best way to grasp the essence of CBT is to combine readings and didactic sessions with opportunities to see therapy being conducted—whether in videos, role plays, or observations of actual sessions. The next step is to practice the methods with patients, ideally with careful supervision from a trained cognitive-behavior therapist. This book has been designed to help you learn CBT in three major ways: reading, seeing, and doing. The videos that accompany the book illustrate key features of CBT. A variety of learning exercises also are provided to help you build skills in implementing cognitive and behavioral techniques.

The video illustrations feature the work of volunteer clinicians who agreed to demonstrate commonly used CBT methods. Videos were filmed in a simple style, because our intent was to show methods that clinicians might use in actual sessions, not to produce slick or professional videos with paid actors following scripts. We wanted to illustrate realistic interventions that have the types of strengths and imperfections characteristic of real treatment sessions. Therefore, we asked four clinicians from varied disciplines to role-play patients with histories and symptoms that were based on cases they had treated. A nurse practitioner, Gina Woods, plays a patient with anxiety disorder (interviewed by the principal author, J.H.W.); a psychiatry resident, Kellye Singletary-Jones, plays a young woman with marital problems and depression (interviewed by another psychiatry resident, Joyce Spurgeon); a psychologist and pastoral counselor, D. Kristan Small, plays a man with depression and anxiety (interviewed by a psychiatrist, Barbara Fitzgerald); and Michael Hollifield, a physician with extensive experience in CBT, plays a man who is having difficulty completing tasks and is experiencing low self-esteem (interviewed by M.E.T., a coauthor of the book).

Instead of showing an entire session for each case, we asked the clinicians to produce brief vignettes (3–10 minutes in duration) that demonstrated key CBT methods such as the collaborative therapeutic relationship, agenda setting, identifying automatic thoughts, examining the evidence, and graded exposure to feared stimuli. This format was chosen because we wanted to illustrate specific points when they occurred in the book and to directly link explanations of core methods with video illustrations. We recommend that you supplement the videos accompanying this book by viewing other taped sessions so that you can see a diverse sample of techniques and styles. Sources for acquiring videos of entire sessions conducted by master cognitive-behavior therapists (e.g., A.T. Beck, Christine Padesky, Arthur Freeman) are listed in Appendix 2, "Cognitive-Behavior Therapy Resources."

The video illustrations are provided on a DVD. To view the videos, place the disc in a DVD player or a computer with a DVD-ROM drive. A menu screen will appear that lists each of the vignettes included on the disc. The videos are intended to be watched in sequence as they appear in the book and at the time you are reading about the specific topic. For example, the first two videos are designed to accompany Chapter 2, "The Therapeutic Relationship: Collaborative Empiricism in Action." We recommend that you wait until you have read the text that explains the methods demonstrated in the videos before viewing them.

When we describe the histories used in the video illustrations, we present them as if they were actual cases. In fact, they are simulations based on amalgams of the clinician's experiences in treating persons with similar problems. We use the convention of describing patients as if they were real throughout the book because of the ease of writing and reading case material with this style of communication. When case material is used, we change genders, background information, and other data so the identities of patients that we or our colleagues have treated are obscured. Also, to avoid the cumbersome phrasing of "he or she," we alternate the genders of personal pronouns when we are not writing about specific cases.

Implementation of CBT can be enhanced by the use of worksheets, checklists, thought records, and other written exercises. Therefore, we have included a number of these helpful forms for you to use in planning or performing CBT. Examples are provided in the text and in Appendix 1, "Worksheets and Checklists." Appendix 1 is also available as a free download in its entirety and in larger format on the American Psychiatric Publishing Web site: http://www.appi.org/pdf/wright.

Specific competencies for performing CBT have been described by the American Association of Directors of Psychiatric Residency Training

(AADPRT). These competencies are discussed in Chapter 11, "Building Competence in Cognitive-Behavior Therapy." However, we elected not to organize the book around these competencies because we wanted to write a guide that would be useful to a broad range of readers, including practicing clinicians and trainees from multiple disciplines. Nonetheless, the book does provide background information and learning exercises that should help psychiatry residents and others acquire the skills described in the AADPRT competencies.

We are indebted to our many teachers and colleagues for their ideas that are incorporated in *Learning Cognitive-Behavior Therapy*. The concepts described in this book are the product of the dedicated work of thousands of researchers and clinicians who have added to the knowledge base of CBT. Our students have also played a large role in our development as educators in CBT. This book is an outgrowth of the courses that we have been teaching at the University of Louisville, the University of Texas Southwestern Medical Center, and the University of Pittsburgh, and of our work together in presenting workshops at meetings of professional organizations. The feedback and suggestions we've received from our students and coworkers have shaped our thinking in many positive directions.

Learning experiences for becoming skilled in CBT can be quite stimulating and productive. Reading about the rich history of CBT can help anchor your treatment interventions to a broad philosophical, scientific, and cultural framework. Studying the theories that underlie the cognitive-behavioral approach can expand your understanding of the psychology of psychiatric disorders and can provide valuable guidance for the practice of psychotherapy. And learning the methods of CBT can give you pragmatic, empirically tested tools for a wide range of clinical problems.

We hope that you will find this book a valuable companion in your work on learning CBT.

Jesse H. Wright, M.D., Ph.D.
Monica R. Basco, Ph.D.
Michael E. Thase, M.D.

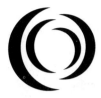

Acknowledgments

Developing a book with video illustrations required a great deal of support from our colleagues, friends, and families. We owe a special note of gratitude to the clinicians (Barbara Fitzgerald, M.D., D. Kristan Small, Ph.D., Michael Hollifield, M.D., Gina Woods, A.R.N.P., Joyce Spurgeon, M.D., and Kellye Singletary-Jones, M.D.) who volunteered to play the therapists and patients in the videos. These clinicians made a major contribution to this book by agreeing to demonstrate CBT skills to a broad audience of readers. The videos were filmed and edited with great care by Randy Cissell from the University of Louisville, and the DVD graphics and navigation system were developed by Rory McMahon from Xerxes, Inc.

Maryrose Manshodi, Christine Johnson, and Theresa King provided invaluable help in manuscript preparation. We also want to express our appreciation to Susanne Wright, D. Kristan Small, Michael Hollifield, Barbara Fitzgerald, and Gina Woods, who read chapter drafts and made astute observations on ways to improve this book. Finally, we want to thank Glen O. Gabbard, M.D., our editor, for his steady guidance and his confidence in our plan to merge text and video in a new volume on learning CBT.

Grant support for the multimedia computer program developed by Jesse H. Wright, M.D., Ph.D., and others and described in this book was received from the National Institute of Mental Health (MH57470), the U.S. Department of Health and Human Services (R41-MH62230), the Norton Community Trust, and the Foundation for Cognitive Therapy and Research.

Disclosure Statement

The principal author, Jesse H. Wright, M.D., Ph.D., may receive a portion of profits from the sale of *Good Days Ahead: The Multimedia Program for Cognitive Therapy* (Wright et al. 2004), described in this book and available at: http://www.mindstreet.com. A portion of profits from sales of this computer program is donated to the Norton Community Trust and the Foundation for Cognitive Therapy and Research.

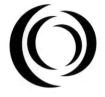

1

Basic Principles of Cognitive-Behavior Therapy

The clinical practice of cognitive-behavior therapy (CBT) is based on a set of well-developed theories that are used to formulate treatment plans and guide the actions of the therapist. This opening chapter focuses on explaining these core concepts and illustrating how the basic cognitive-behavioral model has influenced the development of specific techniques. We begin with a brief overview of the historical background of CBT. The fundamental principles of CBT have been linked to ideas that were first described thousands of years ago (Beck et al. 1979; D.A. Clark et al. 1999).

Origins of CBT

CBT is a commonsense approach that is based on two central tenets: 1) our cognitions have a controlling influence on our emotions and behavior; and 2) how we act or behave can strongly affect our thought patterns and emotions. The cognitive elements of this viewpoint were recognized by the Stoic philosophers Epictetus, Cicero, Seneca, and others two millennia before the introduction of CBT (Beck et al. 1979). For example, the Greek Stoic Epictetus wrote in the *Enchiridion*, "Men are disturbed not by the things which happen, but by the opinions about the things" (Epictetus 1991, p. 14). Also, in Eastern philosophical traditions, such as Taoism and Buddhism, cognition is regarded as a primary force in determining human behavior (Beck et al. 1979; Campos 2002). In his book *Ethics for the New Millennium*, the Dalai Lama (1999) noted, "If we can reorient our thoughts and emotions, and reorder our behavior, not only can we learn to cope with suffering more easily, but we can prevent a great deal of it from starting in the first place" (p. xii).

The perspective that developing a healthy style of thinking can reduce distress or give a greater sense of well-being is a common theme across many generations and cultures. The ancient Persian philosopher Zoroaster based his teachings on three main pillars: thinking well, acting well, and talking well. Benjamin Franklin, one of the founding fathers of the United States, wrote extensively on the development of constructive attitudes, which he believed would favorably influence behavior (Isaacson 2003). During the nineteenth and twentieth centuries, European philosophers—including Kant, Heidegger, Jaspers, and Frankl—continued to develop the idea that conscious cognitive processes play a fundamental role in human existence (D.A. Clark et al. 1999; Wright et al. 2003). For example, Frankl (1992) persuasively argued that finding a sense of meaning in life helped serve as an antidote to despair and disillusionment.

Aaron T. Beck was the first person to fully develop theories and methods for using cognitive and behavioral interventions for emotional disorders (Beck 1963, 1964). Although Beck departed from psychoanalytic concepts, he noted that his cognitive theories were influenced by the work of several post-Freudian analysts, such as Adler, Horney, and Sullivan. Their focus on distorted self-images presaged the development of more systematized cognitive-behavioral formulations of psychiatric disorders and personality structure (D.A. Clark et al. 1999). Kelly's (1955) theory of personal constructs (core beliefs or self-schemas) and Ellis's rational-emotive therapy also contributed to the development of cognitive-behavioral theories and methods (D.A. Clark et al. 1999; Raimy 1975).

Beck's early formulations were centered on the role of maladaptive information processing in depression and anxiety disorders. In a series of papers published in the early 1960s, he described a cognitive conceptualization of depression in which symptoms were related to a negative thinking style in three domains: self, world, and future (the "negative cognitive triad"; Beck 1963, 1964). Beck's proposal for a cognitively oriented therapy targeted at reversing dysfunctional cognitions and related behavior was then tested in a large number of outcome studies (Butler and Beck 2000; Dobson 1989; Wright et al. 2003). The theories and methods outlined by Beck and many other contributors to the cognitive-behavioral model have been extended to a wide array of conditions, including depression, anxiety disorders, eating disorders, schizophrenia, bipolar disorder, chronic pain, personality disorders, and substance abuse. More than 300 controlled studies of CBT have been completed for a variety of psychiatric disorders (Butler and Beck 2000).

The behavioral components of the CBT model had their beginnings in the 1950s and 1960s when clinical researchers began to apply the ideas of Pavlov, Skinner, and other experimental behaviorists (Rachman 1997). Joseph Wolpe (1958) and Hans Eysenck (1966) were pioneers in exploring the potential of behavioral interventions such as desensitization (graded contact with feared objects or situations) and relaxation training. Many of the early approaches to using behavioral principles for psychotherapy paid limited attention to the cognitive processes involved in psychiatric disorders. Instead, the focus was on shaping measurable behavior with reinforcers and extinguishing fearful responses with exposure protocols.

As research on behavior therapy expanded, a number of prominent investigators—such as Meichenbaum (1977) and Lewinsohn and associates (1985)—began to incorporate cognitive theories and strategies into their treatment programs. They noted that the cognitive perspective added context, depth, and understanding to behavioral interventions. Also, Beck advocated the inclusion of behavioral methods from the outset of his work because he recognized that these tools are effective in reducing symptoms and because he conceptualized a close relationship between cognition and behavior. Since the 1960s, there has been a gradual coalescence of cognitive and behavioral formulations for psychotherapy. Although there are still some purists who may debate the merits of using a cognitive or behavioral approach alone, most pragmatically oriented therapists consider cognitive and behavioral methods to be effective partners in both theory and practice.

A good illustration of the coming together of cognitive and behavioral theories can be found in the work of D.M. Clark (1986; D.M. Clark et al. 1994) and Barlow (Barlow and Cerney 1988; Barlow et al. 1989) on treatment programs for panic disorder. They have observed that patients with panic disorder typically have a constellation of cognitive symptoms (e.g., catastrophic fears of physical calamities or loss of control) and behavioral symptoms (e.g., escape or avoidance). Extensive research has demonstrated the efficacy of a combined approach that uses cognitive techniques (to modify fearful cognitions) along with behavioral methods, including breathing training, relaxation, and exposure therapy (Barlow et al. 1989; D.M. Clark et al. 1994; Wright et al. 2003).

The Cognitive-Behavioral Model

The principal elements of the cognitive-behavioral model are diagrammed in Figure 1–1. Cognitive processing is given a central role in this model because humans continually appraise the significance of events in the environment around and within them (e.g., stressful events, feedback or lack of feedback from others, memories of events from the past, tasks to be done, bodily sensations), and cognitions are often associated with emotional reactions. For example, Richard, a man with a social anxiety disorder, was preparing to attend a party in his neighborhood and had the following thoughts: "I won't know what to say....Everyone will know I'm nervous....I'll look like a misfit....I'll clutch and want to leave right away." The emotions and physiological responses that were stimulated by these maladaptive cognitions were predictable: severe anxiety, physical tension, and autonomic arousal. He began sweating, felt "butterflies" in his stomach, and had a dry mouth. His behavioral response was also problematic. Instead of facing the situation and attempting to gain skills in mastering social situations, he called to tell the host that he had the flu.

Avoidance of the feared situation reinforced Richard's negative thinking and became part of a vicious cycle of thoughts, emotions, and behavior that deepened his problem with social anxiety. Each time he maneuvered to escape from social situations, his beliefs about being incapable and vulnerable were strengthened. These fearful cognitions then amplified his emotional discomfort and made it less likely that he would engage in social activities. Richard's cognitions, emotions, and actions are diagrammed in Figure 1–2.

In treating problems like Richard's, cognitive-behavior therapists can draw from a variety of methods that are targeted at all three areas of pathological functioning identified in the basic CBT model: cognitions, emotions, and behaviors. For example, Richard might be taught how to recognize and change his anxiety-ridden thoughts, to use relaxation or imagery to reduce anxious emotions, or to implement a step-by-step hierarchy to break the pattern of avoidance and build social skills.

Before describing theories and methods of CBT in more detail, we want to explain how the model outlined in Figure 1–1 is used in clinical practice and how it relates to broader concepts of the etiology and treatment of psychiatric disorders. The basic CBT model is a construct used to help clinicians conceptualize clinical problems and implement specific CBT methods. As a working model, it is purposefully simplified to direct the attention of the clinician to the relationships among thoughts, emotions, and behaviors and to guide treatment interventions.

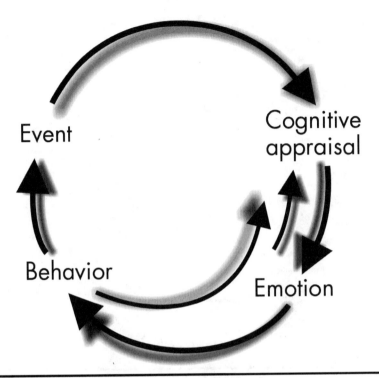

Figure 1–1. Basic cognitive-behavioral model.

Cognitive-behavior therapists also recognize that there are complex interactions among biological processes (e.g., genetics, neurotransmitter functioning, brain structure, and neuroendocrine systems), environmental and interpersonal influences, and cognitive-behavioral elements in the genesis and treatment of psychiatric disorders (Wright 2004; Wright and Thase 1992). The CBT model assumes that cognitive and behavioral changes are modulated through biological processes and that psychotropic medications and other biological treatments influence cognitions (Wright et al. 2003). Recent research has supported this position.

In one study, positron emission tomography (PET) revealed similar findings (of decreased regional cerebral blood flow in brain areas associated with response to threat) in patients who responded to either citalopram or CBT for social phobia (Furmark et al. 2002). In another investigation, normalization of orbitofrontal cortex metabolism on PET scans was positively associated with the degree of improvement in patients with obsessive-compulsive disorder who were treated with behavioral methods or fluoxetine (Schwartz et al. 1996). A study of the biological effects of CBT for depression found cortical activation before

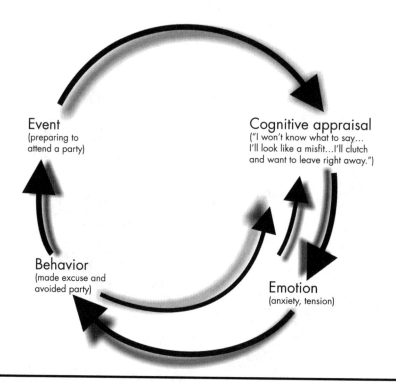

Figure 1–2. Basic cognitive-behavioral model: example of a patient with social phobia.

limbic system stimulation (Goldapple et al. 2004). These findings suggest that biological and cognitive interventions may interact in the treatment of psychiatric disorders.

Research on combined pharmacotherapy and psychotherapy has provided additional support for considering biological influences in implementing the CBT model. Combined treatment with CBT and medication can improve efficacy, especially for severe conditions such as chronic or treatment-resistant depression, schizophrenia, and bipolar disorder (Keller et al. 2000; Lam et al. 2003; Rector and Beck 2001; Wright 2004). However, high-potency benzodiazepines such as alprazolam may impair the effectiveness of CBT (Marks et al. 1993).

To provide overall direction for treatment, an integrated, fully detailed formulation that includes cognitive-behavioral, biological, social, and interpersonal considerations is strongly recommended. Methods for developing multifaceted case conceptualizations are discussed and illustrated in Chapter 3, "Assessment and Formulation." The remainder of this chapter is devoted to introducing the core theories and methods of CBT.

Basic Concepts

Levels of Cognitive Processing

Three primary levels of cognitive processing have been identified by Beck and his colleagues (Beck et al. 1979; D.A. Clark et al. 1999; Dobson and Shaw 1986). The highest level of cognition is *consciousness*, a state of awareness in which decisions can be made on a rational basis. Conscious attention allows us to 1) monitor and assess interactions with the environment, 2) link past memories with present experiences, and 3) control and plan future actions (Sternberg 1996). In CBT, therapists encourage the development and application of adaptive conscious thought processes such as rational thinking and problem solving. The therapist also devotes considerable effort to helping patients recognize and change pathological thinking at two levels of relatively autonomous information processing: *automatic thoughts* and *schemas* (Beck et al. 1979; D.A. Clark et al. 1999; Wright et al. 2003). *Automatic thoughts* are cognitions that stream rapidly through our minds when we are in the midst of situations (or are recalling events). Although we may be subliminally aware of the presence of automatic thoughts, typically these cognitions are not subjected to careful rational analysis. *Schemas* are core beliefs that act as templates or underlying rules for information processing. They serve a critical function in allowing humans to screen, filter, code, and assign meaning to information from the environment.

In contrast to psychodynamically oriented therapy, CBT does not posit specific structures or defenses that block thoughts from awareness (D.A. Clark et al. 1999). Instead, CBT emphasizes techniques designed to help patients detect and modify their inner thoughts, especially those that are associated with emotional symptoms such as depression, anxiety, or anger. CBT teaches patients to "think about their thinking" to reach the goal of bringing autonomous cognitions into conscious awareness and control.

Automatic Thoughts

A large number of the thoughts that we have each day are part of a stream of cognitive processing that is just below the surface of the fully conscious mind. These automatic thoughts are typically private or unspoken and occur in a rapid-fire manner as we evaluate the significance of events in our lives. D.A. Clark and colleagues (1999) used the term *preconscious* in describing automatic thoughts, because these cognitions can be recognized and understood if our attention is drawn to them. Persons with psychiatric disorders such as depression or anxiety often experience floods of automatic thoughts that are maladaptive or distorted. These thoughts can generate painful emotional reactions and dysfunctional behavior.

Event	Automatic thoughts	Emotions
My mother calls and asks why I forgot my sister's birthday.	"I messed up again. There's no way I will ever please her. I can't do anything right. What's the use?"	Sadness, anger
Thinking about a big project that is due at work	"It's too much for me. I'll never get it done in time. I won't be able to face my boss. I'll lose the job and everything else in my life."	Anxiety
My husband complains that I'm irritable all the time.	"He's really down on me. I'm failing as a wife. I don't enjoy anything. Why would anyone want to be around me?"	Sadness, anxiety

Figure 1–3. Martha's automatic thoughts.

One of the most important clues that automatic thoughts might be occurring is the presence of strong emotions. The relationship between events, automatic thoughts, and emotions is illustrated by an example from the treatment of Martha, a woman who was experiencing major depression (Figure 1–3).

In this example, Martha's automatic thoughts demonstrate the common finding of negatively biased cognitions in depression. Although she was depressed and was having problems with her family and her work, she was actually functioning much better than was apparent from her overly critical automatic thoughts. A large body of research has confirmed that persons with depression, anxiety disorders, and other psychiatric conditions have a high frequency of distorted automatic thoughts (Blackburn et al. 1986; Haaga et al. 1991; Hollon et al. 1986; Wright et al. 2003). In depression, automatic thoughts often center on themes of hopelessness, low self-esteem, and failure. Persons with anxiety disorders usually have automatic thoughts that include predictions of danger, harm, uncontrollability, or inability to manage threats (D.A. Clark et al. 1990; Ingram and Kendall 1987; Kendall and Hollon 1989).

Everyone has automatic thoughts; they do not occur exclusively in people with depression, anxiety, or other emotional disorders. By recognizing their personal automatic thoughts and employing other cognitive-behavioral processes, clinicians can improve their understanding of basic concepts, increase their empathy with patients, and deepen awareness of their cognitive and behavioral patterns that could influence the therapeutic relationship.

Throughout this book, we suggest exercises that we believe will help you learn the core principles of CBT. Most of these learning exercises involve practicing CBT interventions with patients or in role-play exercises with a colleague, but in some you will be asked to examine your own thoughts and feelings. The first exercise is to write down an example of automatic thoughts. Try to do this for a situation from your own life. If a personal example does not come to mind, you can use a vignette from a patient you have interviewed.

> **Learning Exercise 1–1.** Recognizing Automatic Thoughts: A Three-Column Thought Record
>
> 1. Draw three columns on a sheet of paper and label them "Event," "Automatic thoughts," and "Emotions."
>
> 2. Now think back to a recent situation (or a memory of an event) that seemed to stir up emotions such as anxiety, anger, sadness, physical tension, or happiness.
>
> 3. Try to imagine being back in this situation, just as it happened.
>
> 4. What automatic thoughts were occurring in this situation? Write down the event, the automatic thoughts, and the emotions on the three-column thought record.

Sometimes automatic thoughts can be logically sound and can be an accurate reflection of the reality of the situation. For example, it could be true that Martha is in danger of losing her job or that her husband is making critical comments about her behavior. CBT does not involve glossing over actual problems. If a person is facing significant difficulties, cognitive and behavioral methods are used to help the person cope with the situation. However, in people with psychiatric disorders, there are usually excellent opportunities to spot errors in reasoning and other cognitive distortions that can be modified with CBT interventions.

Cognitive Errors

In his initial formulations, Beck (1963, 1964; Beck et al. 1979) theorized that there are characteristic errors in logic in the automatic thoughts and other cognitions of persons with emotional disorders. Subsequent research has confirmed the importance of cognitive errors in pathological styles of information processing. For example, cognitive errors have been found to occur substantially more frequently in depressed persons than in control subjects (LeFebvre 1981; Watkins and Rush 1983). Beck and coworkers (1979; D.A. Clark et al. 1999) described six main categories of cognitive errors: selective abstraction, arbitrary inference, overgeneralization, magnification and minimization, personalization, and absolutistic (dichotomous or all-or-nothing) thinking. Definitions and examples of each of these cognitive errors are provided in Table 1–1.

As you probably noticed from reviewing the examples in Table 1–1, there can be a good deal of overlap between cognitive errors. David, the person who was using absolutistic thinking, was also ignoring the evidence of his own strengths and minimizing his friend Ted's problems. The man who fell victim to selective abstraction after not receiving a holiday card had additional cognitive errors such as all-or-nothing thinking ("Nobody cares about me anymore"). In implementing CBT methods for reducing cognitive errors, therapists typically teach patients that the most important aim is simply to recognize that one is making cognitive errors—not to identify each and every error in logic that is occurring.

Schemas

In cognitive-behavioral theory, schemas are defined as basic templates or rules for information processing that underlie the more superficial layer of automatic thoughts (D.A. Clark et al. 1999; Wright et al. 2003). Schemas are enduring principles of thinking that start to take shape in early childhood and are influenced by a multitude of life experiences, including parental teaching and modeling, formal and informal educational activities, peer experiences, traumas, and successes.

Bowlby (1985) and others observed that humans need to develop schemas to manage the large amounts of information that they encounter each day and to make timely and appropriate decisions. For example, if a person has a basic rule of "always plan ahead," it is unlikely that she will spend much time debating the merits of going into a new situation without advance preparation. Instead, she will automatically begin to lay the groundwork for managing a situation.

It has been suggested by D.A. Clark and colleagues (1999) that there are three main groups of schemas:

1. **Simple schemas**

    Definition: Rules about the physical nature of the environment, practical management of everyday activities, or laws of nature that may have little or no effect on psychopathology.

Table 1–1.　Cognitive errors

Selective abstraction (sometimes called *ignoring the evidence* or *the mental filter*)

Definition: A conclusion is drawn after looking at only a small portion of the available information. Salient data are screened out or ignored in order to confirm the person's biased view of the situation.

Example: A depressed man with low self-esteem does not receive a holiday card from an old friend. He thinks, "I'm losing all my friends; nobody cares about me anymore." He ignores the evidence that he has received cards from a number of other friends, that his old friend had sent him a card every year for the past 15 years, that his friend has been busy this past year with a move and a new job, and that he still has good relationships with other friends.

Arbitrary inference

Definition: A conclusion is reached in the face of contradictory evidence or in the absence of evidence.

Example: A woman with a fear of elevators is asked to predict the chances that an elevator will fall if she rides in it. She replies that the chances are 10% or more that the elevator will fall to the ground and that she will be injured. Many people have tried to convince her that the chances of a catastrophic elevator accident are negligible.

Overgeneralization

Definition: A conclusion is made about one or more isolated incidents and then is extended illogically to cover broad areas of functioning.

Example: A depressed college student gets a B on a test. He considers this unsatisfactory. He is overgeneralizing when he has automatic thoughts such as "I'm in trouble in this class; I'm falling short everywhere in my life; I can't do anything right."

Magnification and minimization

Definition: The significance of an attribute, event, or sensation is exaggerated or minimized.

Example: A woman with panic disorder starts to feel light-headed during the onset of a panic attack. She thinks, "I'll faint; I might have a heart attack or a stroke."

Personalization

Definition: External events are related to oneself when there is little or no basis for doing so. Excessive responsibility or blame is taken for negative events.

Example: There has been an economic downturn, and a previously successful business is now struggling to meet the annual budget. Layoffs are being considered. A host of factors have led to the budget crisis, but one of the managers thinks, "It's all my fault; I should have seen this coming and done something about it; I've failed everyone in the company."

Absolutistic (*dichotomous* or *all-or-nothing*) thinking

Definition: Judgments about oneself, personal experiences, or others are placed into one of two categories (e.g., all bad or all good, total failure or total success, completely flawed or completely perfect).

Table 1–1. Cognitive errors *(continued)*

Example: David, a man with depression, compares himself with Ted, a friend who appears to have a good marriage and whose children are doing well in school. Although the friend has a fair amount of domestic happiness, his life is far from ideal. Ted has troubles at work, financial strains, and physical ailments, among other difficulties. David is engaging in absolutistic thinking when he tells himself, "Ted has everything going for him; I have nothing."

    Examples: "Be a defensive driver"; "A good education pays off"; "Take shelter during a thunderstorm."
2. **Intermediary beliefs and assumptions**
    Definition: Conditional rules such as if-then statements that influence self-esteem and emotional regulation.
    Examples: "I must be perfect to be accepted"; "If I don't please others all the time, they will reject me"; "If I work hard, I can succeed."
3. **Core beliefs about the self**
    Definition: Global and absolute rules for interpreting environmental information related to self-esteem.
    Examples: "I'm unlovable"; "I'm stupid"; "I'm a failure"; "I am a good friend"; "I can trust others."

In our clinical practice, we typically do not try to explain the different levels of schemas (e.g., intermediary assumptions vs. core beliefs) to patients. We have found that most patients benefit more from recognizing the general concept that schemas or core beliefs (we use these terms interchangeably) have a strong influence on self-esteem and behavior. We also teach patients that all people have a mixture of adaptive (healthy) schemas and maladaptive core beliefs. Our goal in CBT is to identify and build up the adaptive schemas while attempting to modify or reduce the influence of maladaptive schemas. A short list of adaptive and maladaptive schemas is presented in Table 1–2.

The relationship between schemas and automatic thoughts has been detailed in the *stress-diathesis hypothesis.* Beck and others have suggested that in depression and other conditions, maladaptive schemas may remain dormant until a stressful life event occurs that activates the core belief (Beck et al. 1979; D.A. Clark et al. 1999; Miranda 1992). The maladaptive schema is then strengthened to the point that it stimulates and drives the more superficial stream of negative automatic thoughts. This phenomenon is illustrated in the treatment of Mark, a middle-aged man who became depressed after being laid off from a job.

Table 1–2. Adaptive and maladaptive schemas

Adaptive schemas	Maladaptive schemas
No matter what happens, I can manage somehow.	If I choose to do something, I *must* succeed.
If I work at something, I can master it.	I'm stupid.
I'm a survivor.	I'm a fake.
Others can trust me.	I can never be comfortable around others.
I'm lovable.	Without a man (woman), I'm nothing.
People respect me.	I must be perfect to be accepted.
If I prepare in advance, I usually do better.	No matter what I do, I won't succeed.
There's not much that can scare me.	The world is too frightening for me.

Source. Adapted from Wright et al. 2003.

Mark was not depressed before losing his job, but he began to have many self-doubts after he had trouble finding new work. When Mark looked at the employment section of his local newspaper, he was riddled with automatic thoughts such as "They won't want me"; "I'll never get a job as good as the last one"; "Even if I get an interview, I'll clutch and not know what to say." After starting CBT, the therapist was able to help Mark uncover several deeply held schemas about competence that had hovered below the surface for many years. One of these was "I'm never good enough," a core belief that had been quiescent in better times but was now stimulating a cascade of negative automatic thoughts every time he tried to find a job.

Information Processing in Depression and Anxiety Disorders

In addition to the theories and methods for automatic thoughts, schemas, and cognitive errors, a number of other important contributions have influenced the development of cognitively oriented treatment interventions. We briefly describe some of these research findings on depression and anxiety disorders to provide an expanded theoretical background for treatment methods detailed in later chapters. The key features of pathological information processing in depression and anxiety disorders are summarized in Table 1–3.

The Link Between Hopelessness and Suicide

One of the most clinically relevant findings from research on depression is the association between hopelessness and suicide. A number of studies

Table 1–3. Pathological information processing in depression and anxiety disorders

Predominant in depression	Predominant in anxiety disorders	Common to both depression and anxiety disorders
Hopelessness	Fears of harm or danger	Heightened automatic
Low self-esteem	Increased attention to	information processing
Negative view of	information about	Maladaptive schemas
environment	potential threats	Increased frequency of
Automatic thoughts with	Overestimates of risk in	cognitive errors
negative themes	situations	Reduced cognitive
Misattributions	Automatic thoughts	capacity for problem
Overestimates of negative	associated with danger,	solving
feedback	risk, uncontrollability,	Increased attention to
Impaired performance on	incapacity	self, especially perceived
cognitive tasks requiring	Underestimates of ability	deficits or problems
effort or abstract	to cope with feared	
thinking	situations	
	Misinterpretations of	
	bodily stimuli	

Source. Adapted from Wright et al. 2003.

have demonstrated that depressed persons are likely to have high levels of hopelessness and that lack of hope raises the risk of suicide (Beck et al. 1975, 1985, 1990; Fawcett et al. 1987). Hopelessness was found to be the most important predictor of ultimate suicide in depressed inpatients who were followed up for 10 years after discharge (Beck et al. 1985). Similar findings were described in a related study with outpatients (Beck et al. 1990). Recently, Brown and coworkers (2005) demonstrated that a cognitive-behavioral intervention that includes writing a specific anti-suicide action plan reduces suicide risk.

Attributional Style in Depression

Abramson et al. (1978) and others have proposed that depressed persons assign meanings (attributions) to life events that are negatively distorted in three domains:

1. *Internal versus external.* Depression is associated with a tendency to make attributions to life events that are biased in an internal direction. Thus, depressed individuals commonly take excessive blame for negative events. In contrast, nondepressed persons are more likely to view noxious happenings as being due to external forces such as bad luck, fate, or the actions of others.

2. *Global versus specific.* Instead of viewing negative events as having only isolated or limited significance, people with depression may conclude that these occurrences have far-reaching, global, or all-encompassing implications. Persons who are not depressed have a better capacity to wall off negative events and prevent them from having a pervasive effect on self-esteem and behavioral responses.
3. *Fixed versus changeable.* In depression, negative or troubling situations are viewed as being unchangeable and unlikely to improve in the future. A healthier style of thinking is observed in nondepressed persons, who more often believe that negative conditions or circumstances will recede with time (e.g., "This too will pass").

Research on attributional style in depression has been criticized because early studies were performed with students and nonclinical populations. Other investigations conducted with carefully diagnosed depressed patients have also produced inconsistent results (Wright et al. 2003). Nevertheless, the weight of evidence supports the concept that attributions can be distorted in depression and that CBT methods can be helpful in reversing this type of biased cognitive processing. In our clinical work, we have found that many depressed patients can readily grasp the concept that their thinking style is skewed in the direction of internal, global, and fixed attributions.

Distortions in Response to Feedback

A series of investigations on responses to feedback have revealed differences between depressed and nondepressed persons that have significant implications for therapy. Depressed subjects have been found to underestimate the amount of positive feedback that is given and to expend less effort on tasks after they have been told that they perform poorly (D.A. Clark et al. 1999; DeMonbreun and Craighead 1977; Klein et al. 1976; Loeb et al. 1971; Wenzlaff and Grozier 1988). Nondepressed control subjects have shown patterns that may indicate a *positive self-serving bias*—they may hear more positive feedback than is actually given or downplay the significance of negative feedback (Alloy and Ahrens 1987; Rizley 1978).

Because a goal of CBT is to help patients develop an accurate and rational style of information processing, therapists need to recognize and address possible feedback distortions. One of the principal methods of doing this—providing and asking for detailed feedback in therapy sessions—is described in Chapter 2, "The Therapeutic Relationship: Collaborative Empiricism in Action," and Chapter 4, "Structuring and Educating." These techniques utilize the therapy experience as a learning opportunity for appropriately hearing, responding to, and giving feedback.

Thinking Style in Anxiety Disorders

Persons who experience anxiety disorders have been shown to have several characteristic biases in information processing. One of these areas of dysfunction is a heightened level of attention to information in the environment about potential threats (Mathews and MacLeod 1987). For example, the woman with the elevator phobia described in Table 1–1 may hear creaks or other sounds in an elevator that make her worry about its safety. A person who did not have this fear would probably pay little or no attention to these stimuli. People with anxiety disorders also commonly view the triggers for their fear as being unrealistically dangerous or likely to cause harm (Fitzgerald and Phillips 1991). Many individuals with panic disorder have fears that the panic attacks—or the situations that induce them—may cause catastrophic damage, perhaps even heart attacks, strokes, and death.

Other studies of information processing have shown that patients with anxiety disorders often have a diminished estimate of their ability to manage or cope with fear-laden situations; a sense of uncontrollability; and a high frequency of negative self-statements, misinterpretations of bodily stimuli, and overestimates of the risk for future calamities (Glass and Furlong 1990; Ingram and Kendall 1987; McNally and Foa 1987; Wright et al. 2003). Awareness of these different types of biased information processing can help clinicians plan and implement treatment for anxiety disorders.

Learning, Memory, and Cognitive Capacity

Depression is often associated with significant impairments in ability to concentrate and in performance of challenging, effortful, or abstract learning and memory functions (Weingartner et al. 1981). Reductions in problem-solving capacity and task performance have also been observed in both depression and anxiety disorders (D.A. Clark et al. 1990; Ingram and Kendall 1987). In CBT, these cognitive performance deficits are addressed with specific interventions (e.g., structuring, psychoeducational methods, and rehearsal) designed to enhance learning and assist patients in improving their problem-solving skills (see Chapter 4, "Structuring and Educating").

Overview of Therapy Methods

When clinicians are beginning to learn CBT, they sometimes make the error of viewing this approach as just a collection of techniques or inter-

---

Table 1–4.   Key methods of cognitive-behavior therapy (CBT)

Problem-oriented focus
Individualized case conceptualization
Collaborative-empirical therapeutic relationship
Socratic questioning
Use of structuring, psychoeducation, and rehearsal to enhance learning
Eliciting and modifying automatic thoughts
Uncovering and changing schemas
Behavioral methods to reverse patterns of helplessness, self-defeating behavior, and avoidance
Building CBT skills to help prevent relapse

---

ventions. In doing so, they bypass some of the most important ingredients of CBT and go directly to the implementation of techniques such as thought recording, activity scheduling, or desensitization. It is easy to fall into this trap because CBT is well known for its effective interventions, and patients often like to get involved in specific exercises. However, if you focus prematurely or too heavily on implementing techniques, you will miss the essence of CBT.

Before choosing and applying techniques, you will need to develop an individualized conceptualization that directly ties cognitive-behavioral theories with the patient's unique psychological makeup and constellation of problems (see Chapter 3, "Assessment and Formulation"). The case conceptualization is an essential guide for the work of cognitive-behavior therapists. Other core features of CBT include a highly collaborative therapeutic relationship, artful application of Socratic questioning methods, and effective structuring and psychoeducation (Table 1–4). This book is designed to help you acquire crucial general skills in CBT, in addition to learning specific interventions for common psychiatric conditions. As a prelude to the detailed descriptions in later chapters, we provide a brief overview of treatment methods here.

Therapy Length and Focus

CBT is a problem-oriented therapy that is often delivered in a short-term format. Treatment for uncomplicated depression or anxiety disorders typically lasts from 5 to 20 sessions. However, longer courses of CBT may be necessary if there are comorbid conditions or if the patient has had chronic or treatment-resistant symptoms. CBT for personality disorders, psychosis, or bipolar disorder may need to be extended beyond 20 sessions. In addition, patients with chronic or recurrent illnesses may benefit from a therapy design in which most of the CBT is front-loaded (i.e., there are weekly visits) in the first months of treatment, but the clinician continues to see the patient for intermittent booster sessions for longer periods of time. Psychiatrists who are experienced in this method may use CBT combined with pharmacotherapy in short sessions during the maintenance phase of recurrent depression, bipolar disorder, or other chronic illnesses.

CBT is usually delivered in sessions lasting 45–50 minutes. However, longer sessions have been successfully implemented for rapid treatment of patients with anxiety disorders (Öst et al. 2001). Sessions of less than 50 minutes are usually recommended for inpatients, persons with psychosis, and others with severe symptoms that substantially interfere with concentration (Kingdon and Turkington 2004; Stuart et al. 1997; Wright et al. 1992). Also, as detailed in Chapter 4, "Structuring and Educating," brief sessions of about 25 minutes have been shown to be effective for treatment of depression if combined with a computer-assisted therapy adjunct (Wright et al. 2005). A shortened form of CBT used in combination with a program for a handheld computer has been described for treatment of panic disorder (Newman et al. 1997). Another format for abbreviated therapy sessions is sometimes used by psychiatrists who are experienced in CBT. Brief sessions are employed, along with medications and treatment adjuncts such as computer-assisted therapy and self-help books, as an alternative to the traditional "50-minute hour."

CBT is focused primarily on the here and now. However, a longitudinal perspective—including consideration of early childhood development, family background, traumas, positive and negative formative experiences, education, work history, and social influences—is critical to fully understanding the patient and planning treatment. A problem-oriented approach is emphasized because attention to current issues helps stimulate the development of action plans to counter symptoms such as hopelessness, helplessness, avoidance, and procrastination. Also, cognitive and behavioral responses to recent events are more accessible and verifiable than responses to occurrences in the distant past. An additional benefit of working primarily on current functioning is a reduction in dependence and regression in the therapeutic relationship (Wright et al. 2003).

Case Conceptualization

When we are in CBT sessions and are doing our best work, we sense that the case conceptualization is directly guiding each question, each nonverbal response, each intervention, and the myriad adjustments we make in therapy style to enhance communication with the patient. In other words, we have a carefully thought-out strategy and are not doing therapy by the seat of our pants. As you learn to become an effective cognitive-behavior therapist, you will need to practice developing formulations that bring together information from the diagnostic assessment, observations on the unique background of the patient, and cognitive-behavioral theory in a detailed treatment plan. Case conceptualization methods are detailed in Chapter 3, "Assessment and Formulation."

Therapeutic Relationship

A number of the features of helpful therapeutic relationships are shared between CBT, psychodynamic therapy, nondirective therapies, and other common forms of psychotherapy. These attributes include understanding, kindness, and empathy. Like all good therapists, practitioners of CBT should also have the ability to generate trust and should demonstrate equanimity under pressure. However, in comparison to other well-known therapies, the therapeutic relationship in CBT differs in being oriented toward a high degree of collaboration, a strongly empirical focus, and the use of action-oriented interventions.

Beck and associates (1979) use the term *collaborative empiricism* to describe the patient–therapist relationship in CBT. The patient and therapist work together much as an investigative team, developing hypotheses about the accuracy or coping value of a variety of cognitions and behaviors. They then collaborate on developing a healthier style of thinking, building coping skills, and reversing unproductive patterns of behavior. Cognitive-behavior therapists are typically more active than those who practice other forms of therapy. They help structure sessions, give feedback, and coach patients on how to use CBT methods.

Patients are also encouraged to assume significant responsibility in the treatment relationship. They are asked to give the therapist feedback, to help set the agenda for therapy sessions, and to work on practicing CBT interventions in everyday life situations. Overall, the therapeutic relationship in CBT is characterized by openness in communication and a work-oriented, pragmatic, team-oriented approach to managing problems.

Socratic Questioning

The style of questioning used in CBT is consistent with a collaborative empirical relationship and the goal of helping patients recognize and change maladaptive thinking. *Socratic questioning* involves asking the patient questions that stimulate curiosity and inquisitiveness. Instead of a didactic presentation of therapy concepts, the clinician tries to get the patient involved in the learning process. A specialized form of Socratic questioning is *guided discovery*, in which the therapist asks a series of inductive questions to reveal dysfunctional thought patterns or behavior.

Structuring and Psychoeducation

CBT uses structuring methods such as agenda setting and feedback to maximize the efficiency of treatment sessions, to help patients organize their efforts toward recovery, and to enhance learning. An effort is made to state therapy agendas in terms that give clear direction for the session and permit measurement of progress. For example, well-articulated agenda items might be "develop a plan to get back to work"; "reduce the tension in my relationship with my son"; or "find ways to get over the divorce."

During the session, the therapist guides the patient in using the agenda to productively explore important topics and tries to avoid digressions that have little chance of helping achieve treatment goals. However, therapists have considerable latitude to deviate from the agenda if important new topics or ideas are identified or if staying with the current agenda is not producing the desired results. Regular feedback is given and received by both patient and therapist to check on understanding and to shape the direction of the session.

A variety of psychoeducational methods are used in CBT. Teaching experiences in sessions typically involve using situations from the patient's life to illustrate concepts. Usually the therapist gives brief explanations and follows them with questions that promote the patient's involvement in the learning process. A number of tools are available to assist therapists in providing psychoeducation. Examples are readings in self-help books, handouts, rating scales, and computer programs. A full description of these tools is provided in Chapter 4, "Structuring and Educating."

Cognitive Restructuring

A large part of CBT is devoted to helping the patient recognize and change maladaptive automatic thoughts and schemas. The most frequently used method is Socratic questioning. Thought records are also heavily utilized in CBT. Capturing automatic thoughts on a written form can often kindle a more rational style of thinking.

Other commonly used methods include identifying cognitive errors, examining the evidence (pro-con analyses), reattribution (modifying attributional style), listing rational alternatives, and cognitive rehearsal. The latter technique involves practicing a new way of thinking by imagery or role play. This may be done in treatment sessions with the therapist's assistance. Or, after patients gain experience in using rehearsal methods, they can carry out assignments to practice on their own at home.

The overall strategy of cognitive restructuring is to identify automatic thoughts and schemas in therapy sessions, teach patients skills for changing cognitions, and then have patients perform a series of homework exercises designed to extend therapy lessons to real-world situations. Repeated practice is usually needed before patients can readily modify ingrained, maladaptive cognitions.

Behavioral Methods

The CBT model emphasizes that the relationship between cognition and behavior is a two-way street. The cognitive interventions described above, if successfully implemented, are likely to have salutary effects on behavior. Likewise, positive changes in behavior are typically associated with an improved outlook or other desired cognitive modifications.

Most behavioral techniques used in CBT are designed to help people 1) break patterns of avoidance or helplessness, 2) gradually face feared situations, 3) build coping skills, and 4) reduce painful emotions or autonomic arousal. In Chapter 6, "Behavioral Methods I: Improving Energy, Completing Tasks, and Solving Problems," and Chapter 7, "Behavioral Methods II: Reducing Anxiety and Breaking Patterns of Avoidance," we detail effective behavioral methods for depression and anxiety disorders. Some of the most important interventions that you will learn are behavioral activation, hierarchical exposure (systematic desensitization), graded task assignments, activity and pleasant events scheduling, breathing training, and relaxation training. These techniques can provide you with powerful tools for helping to reduce symptoms and promoting positive change.

Building CBT Skills to Help Prevent Relapse

One of the bonuses of the CBT approach is the acquisition of skills that can reduce the risk for relapse. Learning how to recognize and change automatic thoughts, use common behavioral methods, and implement the other interventions described earlier in this chapter can help patients manage future triggers for the return of symptoms. For example, a person who learns to recognize cognitive errors in automatic thoughts may be better able to avoid catastrophic thinking in stressful situations encountered after therapy ends. During the later phases of CBT, the therapist often focuses specifically on relapse prevention by helping the patient identify potential problems that have a high likelihood of causing difficulty. Then rehearsal techniques are used to practice effective ways of coping.

To illustrate the CBT approach to relapse prevention, consider the case of a person who is being discharged from an inpatient unit after a suicide attempt. Although the individual may be much improved and not currently suicidal, a good cognitive-behavioral treatment plan would include discussion of the possible challenges of return to home and work, followed by coaching on ways to respond to these challenges. It is likely that CBT with this patient also would include the development of a specific antisuicide plan.

Summary

CBT is one of the most widely practiced forms of psychotherapy for psychiatric disorders. This treatment approach is based on precepts about the role of cognition in controlling human emotion and behavior that have been traced to the writings of philosophers from ancient times to the present. The constructs that define CBT were developed by Aaron T. Beck and other influential psychiatrists and psychologists beginning in the 1960s. CBT is distinguished by the large amount of empirical research that has examined its basic theories and has demonstrated the efficacy of treatment.

The learning process for becoming a skilled cognitive-behavior therapist involves studying basic theories and methods, viewing examples of CBT interventions, and practicing this treatment approach with patients. In this chapter, we introduced the core concepts of CBT, such as the cognitive-behavioral model, the importance of recognizing and modifying automatic thoughts, the influence of schemas in information processing and psychopathology, and the key function of behavioral principles in designing treatment interventions. The chapters that follow give detailed explanations and illustrations of how to put the basic principles of CBT to work.

References

Abramson LY, Seligman MEP, Teasdale J: Learned helplessness in humans: critique and reformulation. J Abnorm Psychol 87:49–74, 1978

Alloy LB, Ahrens AH: Depression and pessimism for the future: biased use of statistically relevant information in predictions for self versus others. J Pers Soc Psychol 52:366–378, 1987

Barlow DH, Cerney JA: Psychological Treatment of Panic. New York, Guilford, 1988

Barlow DH, Craske MG, Cerney JA, et al: Behavioral treatment of panic disorder. Behav Ther 20:261–268, 1989

Beck AT: Thinking and depression. Arch Gen Psychiatry 9:324–333, 1963

Beck AT: Thinking and depression, II: theory and therapy. Arch Gen Psychiatry 10:561–571, 1964

Beck AT, Kovacs M, Weissman A: Hopelessness and suicidal behavior—an overview. JAMA 234:1146–1149, 1975

Beck AT, Rush AJ, Shaw BF, et al: Cognitive Therapy of Depression. New York, Guilford, 1979

Beck AT, Steer RA, Kovacs M, et al: Hopelessness and eventual suicide: a 10-year prospective study of patients hospitalized with suicidal ideation. Am J Psychiatry 142:559–562, 1985

Beck AT, Brown G, Berchick RJ, et al: Relationship between hopelessness and ultimate suicide: a replication with psychiatric outpatients. Am J Psychiatry 147:190–195, 1990

Blackburn IM, Jones S, Lewin RJP: Cognitive style in depression. Br J Clin Psychol 25:241–251, 1986

Bowlby J: The role of childhood experience in cognitive disturbance, in Cognition and Psychotherapy. Edited by Mahoney MJ, Freeman A. New York, Plenum, 1985, pp 181–200

Brown GK, Ten Have T, Henriques GR, et al: Cognitive therapy for the prevention of suicide attempts: a randomized controlled trial. JAMA 294:563–570, 2005

Butler AC, Beck JS: Cognitive therapy outcomes: a review of meta-analyses. Journal of the Norwegian Psychological Association 37:1–9, 2000

Campos PE: Special series: integrating Buddhist philosophy with cognitive and behavioral practice. Cognitive and Behavioral Practice 9:38–40, 2002

Clark DA, Beck AT, Stewart B: Cognitive specificity and positive-negative affectivity: complementary or contradictory views on anxiety and depression? J Abnorm Psychol 99:148–155, 1990

Clark DA, Beck AT, Alford BA: Scientific Foundations of Cognitive Theory and Therapy of Depression. New York, Wiley, 1999

Clark DM: A cognitive approach to panic. Behav Res Ther 24:461–470, 1986

Clark DM, Salkovskis PM, Hackmann A, et al: A comparison of cognitive therapy, applied relaxation and imipramine in the treatment of panic disorder. Br J Psychiatry 164:759–769, 1994

Dalai Lama: Ethics for the New Millennium. New York, Riverhead Books, 1999

DeMonbreun BG, Craighead WE: Distortion of perception and recall of positive and neutral feedback in depression. Cognit Ther Res 1:311–329, 1977

Dobson KS: A meta-analysis of the efficacy of cognitive therapy for depression. J Consult Clin Psychol 57:414–419, 1989

Dobson KS, Shaw BF: Cognitive assessment with major depressive disorders. Cognit Ther Res 10:13–29, 1986

Epictetus: Enchiridion. Translated by George Long. Amherst, NY, Prometheus Books, 1991

Eysenck HJ: The Effects of Psychotherapy. New York, International Science Press, 1966

Fawcett J, Scheftner W, Clark D, et al: Clinical predictors of suicide in patients with major affective disorders: a controlled prospective study. Am J Psychiatry 144:35–40, 1987

Fitzgerald TE, Phillips W: Attentional bias and agoraphobic avoidance: the role of cognitive style. J Anxiety Disord 5:333–341, 1991

Frankl VE: Man's Search for Meaning: An Introduction to Logotherapy. Boston, MA, Beacon Press, 1992

Furmark T, Tillfors M, Marteinsdottir I, et al: Common changes in cerebral blood flow in patients with social phobia treated with citalopram or cognitive-behavioral therapy. Arch Gen Psychiatry 59:425–433, 2002

Glass CR, Furlong M: Cognitive assessment of social anxiety: affective and behavioral correlates. Cognit Ther Res 14:365–384, 1990

Goldapple K, Segal Z, Garson C, et al: Modulation of cortical-limbic pathways in major depression: treatment-specific effects of cognitive behavior therapy. Arch Gen Psychiatry 61:34–41, 2004

Haaga DA, Dyck MJ, Ernst D: Empirical status of cognitive theory of depression. Psychol Bull 110:215–236, 1991

Hollon SD, Kendall PC, Lumry A: Specificity of depressotypic cognitions in clinical depression. J Abnorm Psychol 95:52–59, 1986

Ingram RE, Kendall PC: The cognitive side of anxiety. Cognit Ther Res 11:523–536, 1987

Isaacson W: Benjamin Franklin: An American Life. New York, Simon & Schuster, 2003

Keller MB, McCullough JP, Klein DN, et al: A comparison of nefazodone, the cognitive behavioral-analysis system of psychotherapy, and their combination for the treatment of chronic depression. N Engl J Med 342:1462–1470, 2000

Kelly G: The Psychology of Personal Constructs. New York, WW Norton, 1955

Kendall PC, Hollon SD: Anxious self-talk: development of the Anxious Self-Statements Questionnaire (ASSQ). Cognit Ther Res 13:81–93, 1989

Kingdon DG, Turkington D: Cognitive Therapy of Schizophrenia. New York, Guilford, 2004

Klein DC, Fencil-Morse E, Seligman MEP: Learned helplessness, depression, and the attribution of failure. J Pers Soc Psychol 33:508–516, 1976

Lam DH, Watkins ER, Hayward P, et al: A randomized controlled study of cognitive therapy for relapse prevention for bipolar affective disorder: outcome of the first year. Arch Gen Psychiatry 60:145–152, 2003

LeFebvre MF: Cognitive distortion and cognitive errors in depressed psychiatric and low back pain patients. J Consult Clin Psychol 49:517–525, 1981

Lewinsohn PM, Hoberman HM, Teri L, et al: An integrative theory of depression, in Theoretical Issues in Behavior Therapy. Edited by Reiss S, Bootzin R. New York, Academic Press, 1985, pp 331–359

Loeb A, Beck AT, Diggory J: Differential effects of success and failure on depressed and nondepressed patients. J Nerv Ment Dis 152:106–114, 1971

Marks IM, Swinson RP, Basoglu M, et al: Alprazolam and exposure alone and combined in panic disorder with agoraphobia: a controlled study in London and Toronto. Br J Psychiatry 162:776–787, 1993

Mathews A, MacLeod C: An information-processing approach to anxiety. Journal of Cognitive Psychotherapy 1:105–115, 1987

McNally RJ, Foa EB: Cognition and agoraphobia: bias in the interpretation of threat. Cognit Ther Res 11:567–581, 1987

Meichenbaum DH: Cognitive-Behavior Modification: An Integrative Approach. New York, Plenum, 1977

Miranda J: Dysfunctional thinking is activated by stressful life events. Cognit Ther Res 16:473–483, 1992

Newman MG, Kenardy J, Herman S, et al: Comparison of palmtop-computer assisted brief cognitive-behavioral treatment to cognitive-behavioral treatment for panic disorder. J Consult Clin Psychol 65:178–183, 1997

Öst LG, Alm T, Brandberg M, et al: One vs five sessions of exposure and five sessions of cognitive therapy in the treatment of claustrophobia. Behav Res Ther 39:167–183, 2001

Rachman S: The evolution of cognitive behavior therapy, in Science and Practice of Cognitive Behavior Therapy. Edited by Clark DM, Fairburn CG. New York, Oxford University Press, 1997, pp 3–26

Raimy V: Misunderstandings of the Self. San Francisco, CA, Jossey-Bass, 1975

Rector NA, Beck AT: Cognitive behavioral therapy for schizophrenia: an empirical review. J Nerv Ment Dis 189:278–287, 2001

Rizley R: Depression and distortion in the attribution of causality. J Abnorm Psychol 87:32–48, 1978

Schwartz JM, Stoessel PW, Baxter LR Jr, et al: Systematic changes in cerebral glucose metabolic rate after successful behavior modification treatment of obsessive-compulsive disorder. Arch Gen Psychiatry 53:109–113, 1996

Sternberg RJ: Cognitive Psychology. Fort Worth, TX, Harcourt Brace, 1996

Stuart S, Wright JH, Thase ME: Cognitive therapy with inpatients. Gen Hosp Psychiatry 19:42–50, 1997

Watkins JT, Rush AJ: Cognitive response test. Cognit Ther Res 7:125–126, 1983

Weingartner H, Cohen RM, Murphy DL, et al: Cognitive processes in depression. Arch Gen Psychiatry 38:42–47, 1981

Wenzlaff RM, Grozier SA: Depression and the magnification of failure. J Abnorm Psychol 97:90–93, 1988

Wolpe J: Psychotherapy by Reciprocal Inhibition. Stanford, CA, Stanford University Press, 1958

Wright JH: Integrating cognitive-behavioral therapy and pharmacotherapy, in Contemporary Cognitive Therapy: Theory, Research, and Practice. Edited by Leahy RL. New York, Guilford, 2004, pp 341–366

Wright JH, Thase ME: Cognitive and biological therapies: a synthesis. Psychiatr Ann 22:451–458, 1992

Wright JH, Thase ME, Beck AT, et al (eds): Cognitive Therapy With Inpatients: Developing a Cognitive Milieu. New York, Guilford, 1992

Wright JH, Beck AT, Thase M: Cognitive therapy, in The American Psychiatric Publishing Textbook of Clinical Psychiatry, 4th Edition. Edited by Hales RE, Yudofsky SC. Washington, DC, American Psychiatric Publishing, 2003, pp 1245–1284

Wright JH, Wright AS, Albano AM, et al: Computer-assisted cognitive therapy for depression: maintaining efficacy while reducing therapist time. Am J Psychiatry 162:1158–1164, 2005

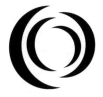

2

The Therapeutic Relationship

Collaborative Empiricism in Action

One of the appealing features of cognitive-behavior therapy (CBT) is the collaborative, straightforward, and action-oriented style of therapeutic relationship that it employs. Although the relationship between therapist and patient is not considered to be the principal mechanism for change as in some other forms of psychotherapy, a good working alliance is a critically important part of treatment (Beck et al. 1979). Just like clinicians of other major schools of psychotherapy, cognitive-behavior therapists seek to provide a treatment environment with a high degree of genuineness, warmth, positive regard, and accurate empathy—the common qualities of all effective therapies (Beck et al. 1979; Keijsers et al. 2000; Rogers 1957). In addition to these nonspecific features of the therapeutic relationship, CBT is characterized by a specific type of working alliance, *collaborative empiricism*, that is geared toward promoting cognitive and behavioral change.

Research on the therapeutic relationship in multiple types of psychotherapy has repeatedly shown a powerful association between treatment outcome and the strength of the therapist–patient bond (Beitman et al. 1989; Klein et al. 2003; Orlinsky et al. 1994; Wright and Davis 1994). A review of investigations of the therapeutic relationship in CBT also revealed that the quality of the cognitive-behavioral therapeutic alliance influences the results of treatment (Keijsers et al. 2000). Particularly notable was the large and influential investigation of a modified form of CBT (the cognitive-behavioral analysis system of psychotherapy; McCullough 2001) for chronic depression; this study demonstrated that measures of the treatment relationship early in therapy predicted subsequent improvement in depressive symptoms (Klein et al. 2003). Thus, there is substantial research evidence that efforts to build therapeutic CBT relationships have a strong impact on the course of treatment.

Learning to forge the most effective therapist–patient relationships is a career-long journey. All clinicians start the process with basic building blocks from their experiences in prior relationships. Among the typical reasons that people choose therapy as a profession is that they have the innate ability to understand others and to discuss emotionally charged topics with considerable sensitivity, kindness, and equanimity. However, learning to maximize these talents usually requires substantial amounts of clinical experience, along with case supervision and personal introspection. As an introduction to the therapeutic relationship in CBT, we briefly discuss the nonspecific features of treatment and then turn to the main focus of this chapter: the collaborative-empirical working alliance.

Empathy, Warmth, and Genuineness

From a cognitive-behavioral perspective, accurate empathy involves the capacity to place yourself in the position of the patient so that you can sense what he is feeling and thinking while retaining objectivity for sorting out possible distortions, illogical reasoning, or maladaptive behavior that may be contributing to the problem. Beck and coworkers (1979) emphasized that it is crucial to properly regulate the amount of empathy and associated personal warmth. If the therapist is perceived as distant, cold, and unconcerned, the prospects for a good treatment outcome will be diminished. However, an overdone effort to be warm and empathic can also backfire. For example, a person with long-standing poor self-esteem or lack of basic trust could perceive an overzealous therapist's attempts to be understanding in a negative light (e.g., "Why should she care so much about a loser like me? The therapist must be lonely herself if she is trying so hard to get to know me. What is the therapist trying to get from me?").

Timing is also very important in making empathic comments. A common mistake is to weigh in heavily with attempts at empathy before patients sense that you adequately understand their plight. However, if you ignore a major display of emotional pain, even in the earliest phases of therapy, you may be seen as disconnected or unresponsive. Here are some good questions to ask yourself as you consider making empathic comments: How well do I understand this person's life circumstances and thinking style? Is this a good time to show empathy? How much empathy is needed now? Are there any risks to being empathic at this time with this patient?

Although well-placed empathic comments usually help strengthen the relationship and relieve emotional tension, there are instances in which attempts to be understanding can reinforce negatively distorted cognitions. For example, if you continually make assurances such as "I can understand the way you feel" to patients who believe that they have failed or their life is unmanageable, you may inadvertently validate their self-condemning and hopeless attitudes. If you are engaged in active listening and are repeatedly nodding your head "yes" while the patient expresses a litany of maladaptive cognitions, she may think that you agree with her conclusions. Or if you have a patient with agoraphobia and you feel so much empathy about the emotional pain of the disorder that you neglect using behavioral methods to break patterns of avoidance, the effectiveness of the therapy may be compromised.

One of the most important keys to showing accurate empathy is genuineness. Therapists who exhibit genuineness are able to communicate verbally and nonverbally in an honest, natural, and emotionally connected manner to show patients that they truly understand the situation. The genuine therapist is diplomatic in giving constructive feedback to patients but does not try to hide the truth. Actual negative events and outcomes are acknowledged as such, but the therapist is always trying to find strengths in patients that will help them cope better with the vicissitudes of life. Thus, one of the desirable personal characteristics of cognitive-behavior therapists is a genuine sense of optimism and a belief in the resilience and growth potential of patients.

Full expression of accurate empathy in CBT includes a vigorous search for solutions. It is not enough to show sensitive concern. The therapist needs to convert this concern into actions that reduce suffering and help the patient manage life problems. Therefore, the cognitive-behavior therapist blends appropriate empathic comments with Socratic questions and other CBT methods that encourage rational thinking and the development of healthy coping behaviors. Often the most effective empathic response involves asking questions that help the patient see new perspectives, instead of simply going along with the flow of a dysfunctional stream of thinking.

Collaborative Empiricism

The term most often used to describe the therapeutic relationship in CBT is *collaborative empiricism*. These two words do a good job of capturing the essence of the treatment alliance. The therapist engages the patient in a highly collaborative process in which there is a shared responsibility for setting goals and agendas, giving and receiving feedback, and putting CBT methods into action in everyday life. Together the therapist and patient target problematic thoughts and behaviors, which are then scrutinized empirically for validity or utility. When actual flaws or deficits are detected, coping strategies for these difficulties are designed and practiced. However, the main job of the therapeutic relationship is to view cognitive distortions and unproductive behavioral patterns through an empirical lens that can reveal opportunities for increased rationality, symptom relief, and improved personal effectiveness.

The collaborative-empirical style of the treatment relationship is illustrated throughout this book in a series of brief videos that demonstrate core CBT methods. We suggest you view two of these vignettes now from Dr. Wright's treatment of Gina, a woman with anxiety disorder. In the first example, Dr. Wright is assessing Gina's symptoms of anxiety and is beginning to plan treatment. Although the therapy has not yet reached the point of specific CBT interventions, therapist and patient are building a solid relationship that will allow them to make progress toward reducing her symptoms of anxiety. In the second example, Gina is being encouraged to take an empirical approach to modifying a set of maladaptive cognitions. A good treatment alliance is an essential requirement for doing this type of therapeutic work.

Before you watch the first video, we want to make a few suggestions on how to get the most out of viewing these demonstrations. As noted in the preface, our goal in producing the video illustrations was to provide examples of how clinicians might implement CBT in actual sessions. The videos were not scripted or designed to be perfect illustrations of the only possible way to treat each situation. Although we asked the clinicians to give the intervention their best effort, and we believe that the videos generally represent solid CBT interventions, you may think of alternative methods or variations in therapy style that may have worked better.

When we show videos in our classes, even when they are sessions conducted by masters such as Aaron T. Beck, we routinely find both strengths and opportunities for doing things differently. Therefore, we recommend that you ask yourself these types of questions when you view the video illustrations in this book: "How did this vignette demonstrate the key principles of CBT?" "What did I like about the therapist's style?"

"What, if anything, would I have done differently?" It also may be useful to view the videos with a colleague or supervisor to compare notes and to generate additional ideas for therapy interventions. Finally, we want to remind you that the videos are designed to be watched in sequence at the point in the book where you are reading about the specific method illustrated in the vignette.

> ▶ **Video Illustration 1.** Assessing Symptoms of Anxiety: Dr. Wright and Gina

> ▶ **Video Illustration 2.** Modifying Automatic Thoughts: Dr. Wright and Gina

Therapist Activity Level in CBT

In addition to the nonspecific relationship qualities common to all effective therapists, cognitive-behavior therapists need to become proficient in demonstrating high levels of activity in treatment sessions. Cognitive-behavior therapists typically work intently at structuring therapy, pacing sessions to get the most out of the available time, developing an ever-evolving case formulation, and implementing CBT methods.

Therapists' activity levels are usually the highest in the early phases of treatment, when patients are more symptomatic and are being socialized to the cognitive-behavioral model. During this part of treatment, the therapist will typically shoulder most of the responsibility for directing the flow of sessions and will spend considerable time explaining and illustrating basic CBT concepts (see Chapter 4, "Structuring and Educating"). The therapist also may need to inject energy, animation, and a sense of hopefulness into the therapy, especially when the patient is severely depressed and is exhibiting pronounced anhedonia or psychomotor slowing. The following case example from the treatment of a depressed man demonstrates how the clinician may sometimes need to be quite active in helping the patient grasp and use CBT methods.

Case Example

Matt was asked to do a thought record for homework after his second session but had trouble completing the assignment.

Therapist: We said that we would spend some time reviewing your homework from last week. How did it go?

Matt: I don't know. I gave it a try, but I was really tired after coming home every night. I never seemed to have enough time to work on it. *(Opens his therapy notebook and takes out the homework.)*

Therapist: Can we take a look at what you wrote on the sheet?
Matt: Sure, but I don't think I did a very good job with it.

The therapist and Matt look at Matt's thought record. The first column has an event ("Wife told me I wasn't fun anymore"); the second column (Thoughts) has no entries; and the third column includes a rating of his feelings ("Sad, 100%").

Therapist: Matt, I can tell that you are getting down on yourself about the homework. Sometimes when people are depressed, it's hard to do this sort of thing. But you did give it a good try, and you did identify a situation that stirred up lots of feelings. If it's all right with you, we can work on completing the other columns here.

Matt (appearing relieved): I was worried that I messed it up and that you would think I wasn't trying.

Therapist: No, I won't judge you. I just want to help you use these types of exercises to get better. Are you ready to talk about what happened when your wife made that remark?

Matt: Yes.

Therapist: I noticed that you wrote down the event and the sad feelings that occurred. But you didn't put anything down in the thoughts column. Can you think back to when your wife told you that you weren't any fun anymore and try to remember what might have been going through your mind?

Matt: It just blew me out of the water. It had been a hard day at work. So, after I came home, I sort of collapsed into my chair and started to read the paper. Then she really laid into me. I guess it upset me so much, I didn't want to write down what I was thinking.

Therapist: That's understandable. I can see that it really upset you. But if we can find out what you were thinking, we may be able to find some clues for ways to fight your depression.

Matt: I can tell you about it now.

Therapist: Let's use this thought record and write down some of the thoughts that you were having at the time. *(Takes thought record and is poised to write.)*

Matt: Well, I guess the first thought was "she's had it with me." Then I started seeing all the important things in my life slipping away.

Therapist: What were you thinking that you were going to lose?

Matt: I was thinking, "She's bound to leave me. I'll lose my family and my kids. My whole life will fall apart."

Therapist: Those are upsetting thoughts. Do you think they are completely accurate? I wonder if depression could be influencing your thinking?

The therapist then explained the nature of automatic thoughts and helped Matt examine the evidence for this stream of negative cognitions. As a result of the intervention, Matt concluded that it was highly likely that his wife was committed to keeping the relationship going but was growing frustrated with his depression. Matt's level of sadness and tension was reduced as the absolutistic nature of his cognitions faded and a behavioral plan was developed to respond to his wife's concerns. This example demonstrates how the therapist may need to take a very active role in explaining concepts, demonstrating central tenets of CBT, and assisting patients to become fully engaged in the treatment process.

You might have noted that the therapist talked more than Matt during much of this interchange. Although there is a great deal of variability from patient to patient and from session to session in how much the therapist will need to talk in CBT, early sessions may be marked by segments with a relatively high level of verbal activity by the therapist. Usually as therapy progresses and patients learn how to use CBT concepts, the therapist will be able to get points across, show empathic concern, and move therapy ahead with fewer words and less effort.

The Therapist as a Teacher-Coach

Do you like to teach? Have you had experiences either being coached or coaching others? Because of the significant importance of learning in CBT, the treatment relationship has more of a teacher–student quality than in most other therapies. Good teacher-coaches in CBT transmit knowledge in a highly collaborative way, using the Socratic method to encourage the patient to be fully involved in the learning process. The following attributes of the therapeutic relationship can promote effective teaching and coaching:

- *Friendly.* Patients typically perceive good therapist-teachers as friendly and kind persons who do not intimidate, prod excessively, or admonish. They convey information in a positive and constructive manner.
- *Engaging.* To be especially effective in the teacher role in CBT, you will need to create a stimulating learning environment. Engage patients with Socratic questions and learning exercises that energize the therapy, but do not overwhelm them with more material or more complexity than they can handle. Emphasize teamwork and the collaborative process in learning.
- *Creative.* Because patients often come to therapy with a fixed, monocular style of thinking, clinicians may need to model more creative ways of viewing the situation and searching for solutions. Try to use learning methods that draw out the patient's own creativity and put these strengths to work in coping with problems.
- *Empowering.* Good teaching usually involves giving patients ideas or tools that allow them to make significant changes in their lives. The empowering nature of CBT is heavily dependent on the educational nature of the therapeutic relationship.

- *Action oriented.* Learning in CBT is not a passive, armchair-style process. Therapist and patient work together to acquire knowledge that is put into action in real-life situations.

Using Humor in CBT

Why should you consider using humor in CBT? After all, most of our patients are facing very serious problems such as the death of loved ones, the breakup of their marriages, medical illnesses, and the ravages of mental illnesses. Could attempts at humor be misconstrued as meaning that you are trying to trivialize, brush off, or ignore the gravity of the patient's problems? Could the patient see your effort to be humorous as a put-down? Is there a chance that the patient will think you are laughing *at* him instead of *with* him?

Of course there are risks in using humor in therapy. Clinicians need to be very careful to recognize potential pitfalls and to gauge the patient's ability to benefit from an injection of humor into the relationship. However, humor can have many positive effects on the patient's ability to recognize cognitive distortions, express healthy emotions, and experience pleasure. For many persons, humor is a highly adaptive coping strategy. It brings emotional release, laughter, and fun into their lives (Kuhn 2002). Yet when patients come to therapy, they often either have lost or have experienced a major decline in their sense of humor.

There are three main reasons to use humor in CBT. First, humor can normalize and humanize the treatment alliance. Because humor is such an important part of life and is often a component of good relationships, judicious and well-placed humorous comments can help promote the friendly, collaborative nature of CBT. The second reason to use humor is to assist patients with breaking out of rigid patterns of thinking and behaving. If the therapist and patient can gently laugh together about the foibles of extreme ways of viewing situations, the patient may be more likely to consider and adopt cognitive changes. The third reason for drawing on the potential of humor in CBT is the possibility that humor skills can be uncovered, strengthened, and enhanced as an important resource for fighting symptoms and coping with stress.

Humor in CBT rarely involves the therapist or the patient cracking jokes. A much more likely scenario involves the use of hyperbole in describing the impact of holding maladaptive beliefs or of persisting with a rigid, ineffective behavioral pattern. Key elements of this type of humor are that it be 1) spontaneous and genuine, 2) constructive, and 3) focused on an external problem or an incongruous way of thinking instead of a personal weakness. Humor that follows these guidelines can loosen the grip of a rigid, dysfunctional set of cognitions or behaviors. Video Illustration 2 includes a number of examples of the therapeutic use of humor in CBT. Dr. Wright and Gina were able to laugh together as they made progress in using the CBT model to attack Gina's anxiety symptoms.

Some therapists are naturally adept at using gentle humor in sessions, whereas others find this aspect of therapy awkward or difficult. Humor is by no means an essential part of CBT. So if you don't like to employ humor or don't have these skills, you can de-emphasize this aspect of therapy and focus on other elements of the collaborative-empirical relationship. However, we still recommend that you ask patients if their sense of humor is one of their strengths and that you help them use their sense of humor as a positive coping strategy.

Flexibility and Sensitivity

Because patients come to treatment with a wide variety of expectations, life experiences, symptoms, and personality traits, therapists need to be attuned to individual differences as they attempt to develop effective working relationships. A monolithic, one-size-fits-all type of therapeutic relationship should be avoided in favor of a flexible, individually tailored style that is sensitive to the unique characteristics of each patient. We suggest that you consider influences from three major domains of clinical interest when customizing treatment alliances: 1) situational issues, 2) sociocultural background, and 3) diagnosis and symptoms (Wright and Davis 1994).

Situational Issues

Current life stresses such as bereavement after the death of a loved one, separation or divorce, job loss, financial problems, or medical illnesses may require adjustments in the therapeutic relationship. An example from our clinical practices is the treatment of a depressed woman who had recently experienced the death of her teenage son from suicide. Because of her profound grief, the therapist needed to make great efforts to be empathic, understanding, and supportive. Typical cognitive-behavioral interventions such as thought recording and examining the evidence were not used in the early part of this treatment because the therapist could better respond to the patient's gaping personal wounds by employing warm concern, active listening, and behavioral interventions to help her resume functioning in everyday life.

Environmental influences or stressors may at times lead patients to make special requests. A patient who is having a troubled marital relationship may ask that bills for therapy not be sent to his home, so that his wife will not know that he is seeing a therapist. A person who has had a surgical complication and is thinking of suing his doctor may stipulate that the surgeon not be contacted to provide medical records. A woman who is involved in a child custody battle may ask the therapist to be her advocate in court. Our general rule for responding to such requests early in therapy is to accept them at face value and to try to meet the patient's expectations unless there is an ethical conflict or professional boundary issue to consider. However, some patients may have expectations that are unrealistic or potentially damaging. Requests, either direct or implicit, for extensive friendship or physical intimacy need to be recognized and managed with firm, ethically responsible guidelines (Gutheil and Gabbard 1993; Wright and Davis 1994). Some other types of requests—such as for extending sessions beyond the normal time frame or for responding to a plethora of phone calls from the patient—may have a negative impact on the alliance. Even though patients can sometimes cite extraordinary situational issues to justify these demands, astute therapists will be aware of the dangers of going overboard in granting special favors.

Sociocultural Background

Sensitivity to sociocultural issues is an essential component of forming authentic and highly functional working alliances. Among other personal variables, gender, ethnicity, age, socioeconomic status, religion, sexual orientation, physical disabilities, and educational level may influence both therapist and patient as they attempt to build a therapeutic relationship. Although clinicians typically seek to be unbiased and to be respectful of diverse backgrounds, beliefs, and behavior, we can have blind spots or lack of knowledge that can interfere with the treatment bond or completely derail our efforts to relate to the patient. Also, patients' biases can significantly impair their ability to benefit from working with therapists whose personal characteristics do not match the patents' expectations.

There are several useful strategies for becoming attuned to the impact of sociocultural influences on the treatment alliance. Our first recommendation is to be introspective in your work with patients from varied backgrounds. Don't assume that you are 100% sensitive to and tolerant of diversity in your patients. Watch closely for negative reactions to patients or evidence that sociocultural factors are limiting your therapeutic efforts. Are you having difficulty expressing empathy with a particular patient? Do you feel stiff or unnatural in treatment sessions? Are you dreading the appointment with this patient? Could any of these responses be due to your personal biases and attitudes? If you spot such reactions, then work out a plan to modify your negative perceptions in order to be more understanding and accepting of the patient.

The second strategy is to make a concerted effort to improve your knowledge of sociocultural differences that can influence the therapeutic relationship. For example, a heterosexual therapist who has limited training about the gay culture and is noticing an aversion to working with homosexual or lesbian patients might read literature about the gay experience, attend workshops designed to improve sensitivity, and view films intended to enhance understanding of issues related to sexual orientation (Spencer and Hemmer 1993; Wright and Davis 1994). Also, clinicians may be able to form more effective alliances if they learn about a wide range of religious traditions and life philosophies. Although a limited amount of research has shown that patients with certain religious beliefs will have an affinity for therapists with similar spiritual backgrounds (Propst et al. 1992), our experiences in using CBT with patients from a variety of religions (or without any specific spiritual leaning) suggest that understanding, tolerance, and respect for different belief structures usually promote good therapeutic alliances.

Clinicians also need to be well versed in ethnic and gender issues that may influence the treatment process (Wright and Davis 1994). In addition to readings and sensitivity training, we suggest that you discuss such issues with experts in cultural diversity and with colleagues and friends to gain a full perspective on these potential influences on the therapeutic relationship. We have particularly valued input from coworkers and associates who have given us feedback about our attitudes. They have helped us deepen our awareness of how ethnicity, gender, and other sociocultural factors can affect the treatment process.

As you are learning more about sociocultural influences on the therapeutic relationship, we also recommend that you take time to examine your office setting for possible biases or slights that may make patients feel uncomfortable. Is the waiting room designed to accommodate persons with physical disabilities or who are grossly overweight? Does the literature in the waiting room convey any particular prejudice? Do office staff members treat all patients with equal respect and attention? Do the decorations of the office convey any unintended meaning that may be off-putting to persons from certain ethnic or cultural backgrounds? If you recognize any features of your office setting that could have a negative impact on therapeutic alliances, then work toward correcting and enhancing the treatment environment.

Diagnosis and Symptoms

Each patient's illness, personality type, and cluster of symptoms can have a substantial influence on the therapeutic relationship. A manic patient may be intrusive and irritating, or he may be overly charming and seductive. Patients with substance use disorders often have cognitive and behavioral patterns that encourage them to deceive the therapist and themselves. A person with an eating disorder can work hard to convince the therapist of the validity of her maladaptive attitudes.

Personality disorders and traits also can have a highly significant effect on the therapist's efforts to establish an effective working alliance. The dependent patient may want to lean on the therapist. A person with obsessive-compulsive personality disorder may have difficulty expressing emotion in therapeutic interchanges. A schizoid patient may be very guarded and have problems trusting the therapist. And of course, a person with borderline personality disorder is likely to have had chaotic and unstable relationships, which can be carried over into the therapeutic arena.

Modifications in CBT methods for specific conditions, including personality disorders, are detailed in Chapter 10, "Treating Chronic, Severe, or Complex Disorders." Here we list three general strategies for managing the impact of the patient's illness and personality structure on the therapeutic alliance:

1. *Spot potential problems.* Be on the lookout for possible influences of symptoms and personality variables, and be ready to adjust your behavior to account for these differences. For example, you may need to pay special attention to developing trust with a person who has been traumatized and is experiencing posttraumatic stress disorder. Or you may want to loosen up, use humor, and try creative approaches to break through the rigidity of a person with obsessive-compulsive traits. If you are treating a woman with an eating disorder whom you suspect is not being fully honest with you about the extent of her unhealthy behavior (e.g., bingeing, purging, abusing laxatives, exercising excessively), open discussions about your concerns may be needed.

2. *Don't label the patient.* Labeling occurs when the clinician slips into using diagnostic terms such as *borderline, alcoholic,* or *dependent* in a pejorative manner. Negative attitudes about these types of behaviors may be subtle, under the surface, or overt. Once labeling occurs, the relationship becomes more distant or strained, the therapist may try less hard to work on symptoms, and the quality of the therapy is likely to deteriorate.

3. *Strive for equanimity.* Try to remain like the calm in the eye of the storm. Be objective and steer a clear course for the therapy, even when you are responding to emotionally charged situations or are challenged by a demanding patient. Work on developing the capacity to deal with a wide

range of clinical situations and personality types while avoiding overreactions, angry behavior, or defensive responses. Your temperament may already contain a healthy dose of equanimity. However, this attribute can be practiced and strengthened. One of the most valuable ways to increase your capacity for equanimity is to build skills in recognizing and managing transference and countertransference reactions, as discussed below.

Transference in CBT

The concept of transference is derived from psychoanalysis and psychodynamic psychotherapy, but it is revised substantially in CBT to be consistent with cognitive-behavioral theories and methods (Beck et al. 1979; Sanders and Wills 1999; Wright and Davis 1994). As in other therapies, transference phenomena are viewed as a reenactment in the treatment relationship of key elements of previous important relationships (e.g., parents, grandparents, teachers, bosses, peers). However, in CBT the focus is not on unconscious components of the transference or on defense mechanisms but on habitual ways of thinking and acting that are recapitulated in the treatment setting. For example, if a man has a deeply held core belief, "I must be in control," and has long-standing behavioral patterns of controlling others, he may play out these same cognitions and behaviors in the therapeutic relationship.

Because CBT is typically a short-term treatment with a straightforward, highly collaborative therapist–patient alliance, the intensity of the transference is usually much lower than in longer-term, dynamically oriented psychotherapy. In addition, transference is not seen as a necessary or primary mechanism for learning or change. Nevertheless, an awareness of transference responses in patients and an ability to use this knowledge to improve treatment relationships and modify dysfunctional thought patterns are important parts of CBT (Beck et al. 1979; Sanders and Wills 1999; Wright and Davis 1994).

In assessing transference in CBT, the therapist watches for schemas and associated behavioral patterns that are likely to have been developed within the context of significant past relationships. This evaluation serves two primary functions. First, the therapist is able to analyze the treatment relationship to learn about the patient's core beliefs and to examine in vivo the effects of these cognitions on the patient's behavior in important relationships. Second, the therapist can design interventions to curtail any negative effects of transference on the treatment bond or on the outcome of therapy.

If there is evidence that a core belief is influencing the therapist–patient relationship, the clinician needs to consider these questions:

1. *Is the transference a healthy or productive phenomenon?* If so, the therapist may elect to withhold any comments about the transference and allow it to continue as is.
2. *Do you think that there is potential for negative effects of the transference?* Perhaps the current state of the transference is neutral or benign, but there is a prospect for complications in the therapeutic relationship. When you spot transference reactions, try to think ahead to what may happen if the therapy keeps going and the relationship intensifies. Preventive actions (e.g., setting strict boundaries, detailing appropriate guidelines for the treatment alliance) may help avoid future problems.
3. *Is there a transference reaction that needs attention now?* When there is a transference reaction that is interfering with the collaboration, is blocking progress, or is having a destructive effect on the therapy, the therapist needs to take prompt action to address the problem. Interventions may include psychoeducation on the transference phenomenon, use of standard CBT techniques to modify automatic thoughts and schemas involved in the transference, behavioral rehearsal (practicing alternate, healthier behaviors in therapy sessions), and contracting to limit or stop certain behaviors.

Case Example

The treatment of Carla, a 25-year-old woman with severe depression, by a middle-aged, female therapist included work on bringing a transference reaction to light and using the transference to help the patient change. The patient's core beliefs (e.g., "I can never be a competent person"; "I'll never be able to satisfy my parents"; "I'm a failure") were negatively affecting the relationship because the patient was comparing herself to the therapist, a successful professional. Carla was also having automatic thoughts that the therapist was judging her and was thinking that she was lazy or dull because she was not always able to show success in implementing CBT self-help methods. As a result, Carla felt distant from the therapist and perceived her as a demanding person who didn't like her very much.

The therapist recognized that Carla's experiences of having hypercritical parents and always believing that she was inferior to others had set her up for having a strained therapeutic relationship. Therefore, the therapist openly discussed the transference reaction and then used CBT methods to correct distortions that were impairing the collaborative bond.

Some of the specific cognitions about the therapist that were targeted for change were the following: "She has everything going for her—I have nothing" (an automatic thought with a cognitive error: maximizing the positives of others and minimizing one's own strengths); "If she really got to know me, she would realize I'm a fraud" (a maladaptive schema that was driving a wedge between the patient and the therapist); and "I could never measure up to her standards" (a transference of beliefs about parents to the therapist).

After eliciting these cognitions, the therapist explained how automatic thoughts, core beliefs, and behaviors from other relationships can be re-enacted in therapy and in other current interpersonal situations. Then she reassured Carla that she understood and respected her, but wanted to help build her self-esteem. They agreed that one way to improve Carla's self-image would be to talk regularly about the therapy alliance and to test out her assumptions about the therapist's attitudes and expectations. As treatment progressed, the therapeutic relationship became a healthy mechanism for Carla to see herself accurately and to develop more realistic, functional attitudes.

Countertransference

Another responsibility of cognitive-behavior therapists is to look for possible countertransference reactions that may be interfering with the development of collaborative treatment relationships. Countertransference occurs in CBT when the relationship with the patient activates automatic thoughts and schemas in the clinician, and these cognitions have the potential for influencing the therapy process. Because automatic thoughts and schemas can operate outside your full awareness, a good way to spot possible countertransference reactions is to recognize emotions, physical sensations, or behavioral responses that may be stimulated by your cognitions. Common indicators that countertransference may be occurring are that you feel angry, tense, or frustrated with the patient; are becoming bored in the therapy; are relieved when the patient is late or cancels the appointment; have repeated difficulties working with a particular type of illness, symptom cluster, or personality dimension; or are finding yourself particularly attracted or drawn to a certain patient.

When you suspect that countertransference may be developing, you can apply the theories and methods of CBT described throughout this book to better understand and manage the reaction. Begin by trying to identify your automatic thoughts and schemas. Then if it is clinically indicated and feasible, you can work on modifying the cognitions. For example, if you have automatic thoughts such as "This patient has no motivation...all he does is whine through the entire session...this therapy is going nowhere," you can try to spot your cognitive errors (e.g., all-

or-nothing thinking, ignoring the evidence, jumping to conclusions) and change your thinking to reflect a more balanced view of the patient's efforts and potential.

Summary

An effective alliance between therapist and patient is an essential condition for implementation of the specific methods of CBT. As therapists engage patients in the process of CBT, they need to show understanding; appropriate empathy and personal warmth; and flexibility in responding to the unique features of each person's symptoms, beliefs, and sociocultural background. Good therapeutic relationships in CBT are characterized by a high degree of collaboration and an empirical style of questioning and learning. The collaborative-empirical treatment alliance brings the therapist and patient together in a joint effort to define problems and search for solutions.

References

Beck AT, Rush AJ, Shaw BF, et al: Cognitive Therapy of Depression. New York, Guilford, 1979

Beitman BD, Goldfried MR, Norcross JC: The movement toward integrating the psychotherapies: an overview. Am J Psychiatry 146:138–147, 1989

Gutheil TG, Gabbard GO: The concept of boundary in clinical practice: theoretical and risk-management dimensions. Am J Psychiatry 150:188–196, 1993

Keijsers GP, Schaap CP, Hoogduin CAL: The impact of interpersonal patient and therapist behavior on outcome in cognitive-behavior therapy: a review of empirical studies. Behav Modif 24:264–297, 2000

Klein DN, Schwartz JE, Santiago NJ, et al: Therapeutic alliance in depression treatment: controlling for prior change and patient characteristics. J Consult Clin Psychol 71:997–1006, 2003

Kuhn C: The Fun Factor: Unleashing the Power of Humor at Home and on the Job. Louisville, KY, Minerva Books, 2002

McCullough JP Jr: Skills Training Manual for Diagnosing and Treating Chronic Depression: Cognitive Behavioral Analysis System of Psychotherapy. New York, Guilford, 2001

Orlinsky D, Grawe K, Parks B: Process and outcome in psychotherapy—noch einmal, in Handbook of Psychotherapy and Behavior Change, 4th Edition. Edited by Bergin AE, Garfield SL. New York, Wiley, 1994, pp 270–376

Propst LR, Ostrom R, Watkins P, et al: Comparative efficacy of religious and nonreligious cognitive-behavioral therapy for the treatment of clinical depression in religious individuals. J Consult Clin Psychol 60:94–103, 1992

Rogers CR: The necessary and sufficient conditions of therapeutic personality change. J Consult Clin Psychol 21:95–103, 1957

Sanders D, Wills F: The therapeutic relationship in cognitive therapy, in Understanding the Counselling Relationship: Professional Skills for Counsellors. Edited by Feltham C. Thousand Oaks, CA, Sage, 1999, pp 120–138

Spencer S, Hemmer R: Therapeutic bias with gay and lesbian clients: a functional analysis. The Behavior Therapist 16:93–97, 1993

Wright JH, Davis D: The therapeutic relationship in cognitive-behavioral therapy: patient perceptions and therapist responses. Cognitive and Behavioral Practice 1:25–45, 1994

Assessment and Formulation

The process of evaluating patients for cognitive-behavior therapy (CBT) and performing case conceptualizations is based on a comprehensive treatment model. Although the cognitive and behavioral elements of understanding the patient's illness are given the greatest emphasis, biological and social influences are also considered to be essential features of the assessment and formulation. In this chapter, we discuss indications for CBT, patient characteristics that are associated with an affinity for this approach, and key dimensions of assessing suitability for therapy. We also introduce a pragmatic method for organizing case conceptualizations and developing treatment plans.

Assessment

An assessment for CBT starts with the fundamental features of evaluation for any form of psychotherapy: a full history and mental status ex-

---

The case formulation worksheet mentioned in this chapter, located in Appendix 1, "Worksheets and Checklists," is also available as a free download in a larger format on the American Psychiatric Publishing Web site: http://www.appi.org/pdf/wright.

amination. Attention should be paid to the patient's current symptoms, interpersonal relationships, sociocultural background, and personal strengths, in addition to consideration of the impact of developmental history, genetics, biological factors, and medical illnesses. A detailed evaluation of influences from these multiple domains will allow you to produce a multifaceted case formulation, as detailed in the next section, "Case Conceptualization in CBT."

Because the indications for CBT are based largely on diagnosis, completion of a standard interview and multiaxial diagnosis will provide much of the information needed to assess the patient's suitability for CBT. Since the 1980s, the CBT model of therapy has been adapted and modified for a large range of conditions, greatly broadening its scope beyond treatment of mild to moderate depressive and anxiety disorders (Wright et al. 2003). For example, in Chapter 10, "Treating Chronic, Severe, or Complex Disorders," we review modifications of CBT for bipolar disorder, schizophrenia, borderline personality disorder, and other conditions that are difficult to treat. We therefore suggest that most of the patients whom you evaluate for psychiatric treatment will be potential candidates for CBT, either alone or in combination with appropriate pharmacotherapy.

CBT is the best-studied form of psychotherapy (Butler and Beck 2000; Dobson 1989; Wright et al. 2003). The efficacy of CBT for a variety of Axis I disorders has been demonstrated in more than 300 randomized, controlled trials (Butler and Beck 2000). Efficacy as monotherapy (i.e., without concomitant pharmacotherapy) has been established for a number of conditions, and CBT is considered one of the treatments of first choice for major depressive disorder, anxiety disorders, bulimia nervosa, and several other conditions (Wright et al. 2003). Although CBT is not an appropriate monotherapy for patients with schizophrenia or bipolar disorder, it has been demonstrated to have utility for these problems when combined with pharmacotherapy (Lam et al. 2003; Rector and Beck 2001; Sensky et al. 2000; see Chapter 10, "Treating Chronic, Severe, or Complex Disorders"). Also, a modified form of CBT has been shown to be useful in borderline personality disorder (Linehan et al. 1991), and treatment methods have been described for other Axis II conditions (Beck and Freeman 1990) and substance use disorders (Beck et al. 1993; Thase 1997).

There are few absolute contraindications for use of CBT (e.g., advanced dementia, other severe amnestic disorders, and more transient confusional states such as delirium or drug intoxication). Persons with severe antisocial personality disorder, malingering, or other conditions that markedly impair the development of a collaborative and trusting therapeutic relationship are also poor candidates for CBT. The factors that limit use of CBT in these conditions apply to other forms of psychotherapy as well.

We discuss the use of longer-term models of CBT to treat patients with more severe disorders or other complex conditions in Chapter 10, "Treating Chronic, Severe, or Complex Disorders." Our focus in this chapter is on identifying the types of patients for whom CBT can be expected to work within a 2- to 4-month time frame. For this purpose, we have drawn from earlier contributions on brief psychodynamic psychotherapy (Davanloo 1978; Malan 1973; Sifneos 1972) and from the thoughtful work of Safran and Segal (1990). Safran and Segal developed a semistructured interview to assess patients' suitability for time-limited CBT. Although this interview has excellent psychometric characteristics, the Safran and Segal method is impractical for use outside of research settings because it takes 1–2 hours to complete. The recommendations we make here are derived in part from Safran and Segal's contributions but are designed to be integrated into the initial evaluation as part of the standard psychiatric assessment.

Who are the ideal candidates for treatment with CBT alone? To some extent, time-limited CBT is best suited for the prototypically easy-to-treat person (i.e., an adult in good health with relatively acute anxiety or a nonpsychotic depressive disorder, who has good verbal skills and some past success in relationships and who is motivated to make use of therapy). Of course, such individuals probably have the best chance of responding to any form of professional intervention or, for that matter, a greater likelihood of remitting spontaneously without any treatment. To these generic good-prognosis indicators we would add factors such as adequate financial resources, safe housing, and supportive family members or close friends. Fortunately, there is good evidence that the utility of CBT is *not* limited only to the easy to treat. Several additional dimensions of suitability for time-limited therapy are discussed below (Table 3–1).

Table 3–1. Dimensions to consider in evaluating patients for cognitive-behavior therapy

---

Chronicity and complexity
Optimism about the chances of success in therapy
Acceptance of responsibility for change
Compatibility with the cognitive-behavioral rationale
Ability to access automatic thoughts and identify accompanying emotions
Capacity to engage in a therapeutic alliance
Ability to maintain and work within a problem-oriented focus

The first dimension noted in Table 3–1 is a general prognostic indicator: the *chronicity and complexity* of the patient's problems. You should adhere to the basic wisdom that long-standing problems typically warrant longer courses of therapy; the same can be said for treatment of depressive or anxiety disorders that are complicated by substance abuse, significant personality disorders, a history of early trauma or neglect, or other comorbid conditions (see Chapter 10, "Treating Chronic, Severe, or Complex Disorders"). The patient's treatment history may provide important clues about the treatability of his or her condition. If you are the twelfth therapist in 25 years or are being asked to try a new approach after the failure of extensive courses of pharmacotherapy and psychotherapy, the appropriateness of offering a 12- or 16-week treatment program could be called into question.

The second dimension, *optimism about the chances of success in therapy*, is also a global prognostic indicator, both for helping relationships in general (Frank 1973) and for CBT in particular (Mercier et al. 1992). There are two pathways by which high levels of pessimism can diminish a patient's ability to respond to therapy. On the one hand, pessimism can reflect a patient's valid assessment that he or she has serious difficulties, particularly when there has been a history of prior unsuccessful courses of treatment. Depression does tend to remove the common tendency of people to minimize their problems and overvalue their strengths. On the other hand, demoralization can undercut the patient's capacity to engage in therapeutic exercises or, through a self-fulfilling prophecy, can discount evidence of progress. Because pessimism is associated with both hopelessness and suicidal ideation, you should be vigilant to the possibility that in some patients a marked level of pessimism may warrant alternate therapies or even hospitalization. In the most extreme sense, pessimism may conceal nihilistic delusions, which indicate the need for antipsychotic medication.

The third dimension, *acceptance of responsibility for change*, is linked to the model of motivation described by Prochaska and DiClemente (1992). Although originally used for assessing persons with substance abuse, this approach is increasingly being applied in other treatment settings. Ask yourself these questions: Why has this person come for treatment? What does he want to accomplish? How much does he want to exert his personal efforts in the change process? Then guide your interview from the general (e.g., "What is your understanding about the causes of depression?" or "What role do you think is best for the patient to play in therapy?") to more specific questions about CBT (e.g., "Based on what you know about panic disorder, what are your impressions about the type of treatment that might work best for you?"). Patients who believe that their condition is caused by a hormonal disturbance or a chemical imbalance may be less than enthusiastic about CBT. Patients who express strong preferences for a medical model of treatment ("I'd really rather just take medicine, but my primary care doctor sent me here because she thinks that therapy is a better solution") likewise tend to be more skeptical of their prospects for psychotherapy. Conversely, persons who are ready to change and express genuine interest in looking at psychosocial influences on symptoms may be more likely to accept and benefit from CBT.

The fourth dimension of the assessment is closely related to the third; *compatibility with the cognitive-behavioral rationale* concerns the specific impressions of both the patient and the therapist about the appropriateness of CBT. Just as in everyday life, first impressions are important; in fact, two studies have shown that patients who gave CBT high marks before beginning therapy responded significantly better than patients who had more neutral or negative initial impressions (Fennell and Teasdale 1987; Shaw et al. 1999). Another specific aspect of compatibility is the willingness to perform self-help exercises or homework. As we emphasize throughout this book, homework is an essential and defining component of CBT. There is ample evidence that patients who do not regularly complete homework assignments are significantly less likely to respond to therapy than those who do (Bryant et al. 1999; Thase and Callan, in press).

Interestingly, though, compatibility does not mean that the patient must have thinking processes loaded with logical errors and cognitive distortions. Whereas novice therapists often think that patients who report a high level of dysfunctional negative thinking are perfect candidates for CBT, there is fairly consistent evidence that such patients do not respond as well as those with less extreme levels of cognitive disturbance (see, for example, Whisman 1993). You may find it more useful to work from the perspective that CBT capitalizes on patients' strengths, rather than trying to correct or overcome their more pronounced weaknesses (Rude 1986). Consistent with this view, severely depressed patients with higher levels of learned resourcefulness (the tendency to think that problems have solutions and to use active methods of problem solving) responded better to CBT than patients with lower levels of learned resourcefulness (Burns et al. 1994).

Although extreme pessimism and markedly high levels of dysfunctional attitudes have potentially negative prognostic implications, the fifth dimension, *ability to access automatic thoughts and identify accompanying emotions*, reflects a real aptitude for CBT. Staying with the view that therapy builds on strengths, you will find that patients who are able to identify and speak aloud their negative automatic thoughts during periods of depressed or anxious mood typically can begin to use three- and five-column exercises earlier in the course of therapy. As a means to help uncover automatic negative thoughts, it can be useful in the initial evaluation to ask the patient about the thoughts and associated feelings she had while she was driving to the session or sitting in the waiting room. Questions to further probe the patient's ability to identify and express negative automatic thoughts (e.g., "What were you thinking during that situation?" or "What thoughts ran through your mind when you were feeling so blue?") are also typically used in assessing suitability for CBT. Difficulty with identifying fluctuations in emotional states is a disadvantage in CBT because patients will miss opportunities to identify *hot thoughts* (i.e., automatic negative thoughts experienced in concert with strong emotional states) and to practice ways of improving mood with cognitive restructuring methods.

The sixth relevant dimension in assessing suitability for short-term therapy deals with the patient's *capacity to engage in a therapeutic alliance.* Safran and Segal (1990) suggested that both observations about behavior in sessions and questions about the patient's history of intimate relationships can provide important clues about his ability to form an effective treatment relationship. During the initial session, direct solicitation of feedback (e.g., "How do you feel about today's session?") and observations about the patient's ability to *connect* (e.g., eye contact, posture, and degree of comfort related to the therapist) are used to gauge capacity to engage in a helping alliance. Historical questions pertaining to the quality of relationships with parents, siblings, teachers, coaches, and romantic partners can provide useful information—particularly when repetitive patterns of disappointment, rejection, or exploitation are revealed. Likewise, if the patient has prior experiences with psychotherapy, his impressions about the quality of that dyad are likely to convey some information about what the future might hold in store.

The seventh and final dimension to be considered is the patient's *ability to maintain and work within a problem-oriented focus.* From the perspective of Safran and Segal (1990), this dimension has two components: *security operations* and *focality.* The former refers to the patient's use of potentially therapy-disrupting behaviors to restore a sense of emotional security when psychologically threatened. Examples are 1) attempts to overly control the pace or topics of conversation during the interview, 2) avoidance of emotionally charged material, or 3) use of long-winded (and tangential) discourse. *Focality,* by contrast, refers to the capacity to work within the structure of CBT sessions and to maintain attention on a relevant topic from start to finish.

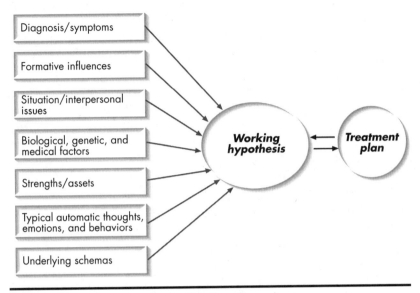

Figure 3–1. Case conceptualization flow chart.

Case Conceptualization in CBT

The case conceptualization, or formulation, is a road map for your work with the patient. It brings together information from seven key domains: 1) diagnosis and symptoms; 2) contributions of childhood experiences and other formative influences; 3) situational and interpersonal issues; 4) biological, genetic, and medical factors; 5) strengths and assets; 6) typical patterns of automatic thoughts, emotions, and behaviors; and 7) underlying schemas (Figure 3–1). In short, all of the important findings from your assessment of the patient are considered in developing a case formulation.

At first glance, it may seem to be a daunting task to synthesize all this information in devising a specific plan for an individual patient. However, the system we describe in this chapter will give you a pragmatic and easy-to-use method for organizing case formulations. The pivotal step in conceptualizing a case is the formation of a working hypothesis (see Figure 3–1). The clinician uses cognitive-behavioral constructs to develop an individualized theoretical formulation relevant to the patient's particular blend of symptoms, problems, and resources. This working hypothesis is then used to direct treatment interventions.

Early in therapy, the case conceptualization may be just an outline or a sketch. You may be uncertain about the diagnosis or you may still be collecting critical parts of the data. You also might have just started to try some CBT interventions. However, it is vital to begin to think about the formulation from the very beginning of treatment. As you get to know the patient better, more observations and layers of complexity can be added to the formulation. You will be able to test your theories to see if they are accurate, and you will learn if your treatment methods are on target. If not, the formulation will need to be revised. For example, if you begin to recognize long-standing dependent features that are stalling progress, you will need to consider altering the treatment plan. If previously unrecognized strengths become apparent, the course of therapy can be changed to take advantage of these assets.

By the middle and late phases of CBT, the case conceptualization should mature to a well-orchestrated plan that provides a coherent and effective guide for each therapy intervention. If you reviewed a taped session from this part of therapy and stopped the tape at any juncture, you should be able to explain your rationale for following the path you are taking at that moment and for the entire course of therapy. Ideally, you would also be able to describe the obstacles to be faced in achieving the best results and a plan for overcoming these obstacles.

The system that we recommend for developing case conceptualizations is based on guidelines established by the Academy of Cognitive Therapy. This organization's Web site (http://www.academyofct.org) contains detailed instructions for writing formulations that meet standards for certification in cognitive therapy. Case examples are also provided. We have distilled the main features of the Academy of Cognitive Therapy case conceptualization guidelines into a case formulation worksheet (Figure 3–2; see also Appendix 1, "Worksheets and Checklists," for blank copies of this form).

To complete the CBT case formulation worksheet, you will need to be able to perform a thorough assessment, as described in this chapter, and you will need to know the core theories and methods of CBT. Because you may not yet be armed with all the information and skills required for developing fully realized case conceptualizations, our goal at this point in the book is modest. We want to introduce formulation methods and to give some examples that will show how CBT constructs can be used in planning treatment. As you work your way through the rest of the book and gain additional experience in CBT, you can build expertise in performing case conceptualizations.

Figure 3–2 shows a case formulation worksheet that Dr. Wright developed for the treatment of Gina, the middle-aged woman with anxiety disorder featured in the video illustrations.

Patient Name: Gina

Diagnoses/Symptoms: Panic disorder with agoraphobia, elevator phobia. Primary symptoms are panic attacks, tension, hyperventilation, and avoidance.

Formative Influences: Grandmother became ill and died when Gina was 7; older sister had congenital heart disease and was told to avoid stress; mother was tense and gave the message that the world was a very dangerous place.

Situational Issues: New job requires driving through heavy traffic; fiancé is now driving Gina to work.

Biological, Genetic, and Medical Factors: Mother had chronic anxiety but did not receive treatment.

Strengths/Assets: Intelligent, articulate, good sense of humor, support from fiancé and family.

Treatment Goals: 1) Reduce panic attacks to one a week or less, 2) be able to go to crowded places (e.g., cafeteria) without having a panic attack, 3) be able to ride elevators, and 4) drive "wherever I want to go."

Event 1	Event 2	Event 3
Going to a crowded cafeteria	Thinking of riding in an elevator	Thinking of driving myself to work
Automatic Thoughts	**Automatic Thoughts**	**Automatic Thoughts**
"I'll drop my tray." "I'll faint." "I'll die."	"The elevator will fall." "It will be crowded." "I'll get stuck."	"I'll faint when I'm driving." "I'll have a wreck." "I'll kill someone on the highway."
Emotions	**Emotions**	**Emotions**
Anxiety, panic, sweating hands, fast breathing	Anxiety, tension, fast breathing	Anxiety, tension, sweating, fast breathing
Behaviors	**Behaviors**	**Behaviors**
Avoid the cafeteria or ask a friend to go along.	Take the stairs if possible.	Don't drive. Ask fiancé to drive.

Schemas: "I'm bound to be hurt"; "I'm the one who will be in an accident"; "The world is a very dangerous place"; "You must always protect yourself."

Figure 3–2. Case formulation worksheet for Gina.

Working Hypothesis: 1) Gina has unrealistic fears of situations, underestimates her ability to control or manage these situations, and avoids the feared stimuli. 2) Her family background (e.g., illnesses and death, mother's tension and hypervigilance) contributed to the development of anxiety-ridden schemas and avoidance. 3) Current situational factors (new job and pressure to drive) may have played a role in triggering symptoms.

Treatment Plan: 1) Cognitive restructuring (e.g., examining the evidence, spotting cognitive errors, using thought records) to teach Gina that her fears are unrealistic and that she can learn to cope with her anxieties; 2) breathing training and imagery to provide tools for controlling anxiety; 3) graded exposure to feared stimuli (e.g., crowds, driving); 4) in vivo exposure for the elevator phobia; 5) modeling and coaching on ways to manage anxiety; and 6) later in therapy, focusing on revising maladaptive schemas.

Figure 3–2.   Case formulation worksheet for Gina.

Case Example

Gina described a host of anxiety-related symptoms, including panic attacks, hyperventilation, sweating, and avoidance of feared situations (e.g., being in crowds, eating in public places, driving, and riding in elevators). She gave a history of having these symptoms for more than 3 years. There was no clear precipitant, but she noted that the anxiety began to increase after she took a new job that required her to drive through heavy traffic to go into the city and to work in a busy office building.

Several formative influences from Gina's earlier years appeared to have shaped her vulnerability to anxiety symptoms. Gina was the second of two children raised in a loving family environment with both parents present in the home. Although she did not report any specific childhood traumas, Gina did have memories from about age 7 of her grandmother coming home from the hospital after a cancer operation. Her grandmother was so ill that she could no longer take care of herself, so she stayed at Gina's house until she died about 6 months later. Gina recalled that her grandmother was in considerable pain and would often cry at night. In addition, Gina's mother was on edge during this illness and for many years afterward.

Gina's view of the world was also influenced by having an older sister with congenital heart disease. Her sister was always told by her parents to be very careful not to overextend herself and to avoid stress. Gina's mother was described as a worrywart. She was especially concerned about Gina during the time when Gina was learning to drive, and she gave Gina repeated instructions to be careful because of the high risk of an accident among teenage drivers. Although her mother never received treatment for anxiety, she was a tense woman who appeared to be excessively concerned about danger and gave her two daughters the message that the world is a very risky place.

Fortunately, Gina had a number of strengths that could be tapped in the process of doing CBT. She was genuinely interested in learning about CBT and was willing to engage in exposure therapy—a key element of CBT for anxiety disorders. She was articulate and intelligent and had a good sense of humor. She was also free of Axis II problems and had excellent support from her fiancé and family members. However, she had long-standing anxiety symptoms with well-entrenched patterns of avoidance, which were likely to require extensive CBT work before resolution. It also appeared that her fiancé, coworkers, and friends were unknowingly reinforcing the anxiety by participating in her elaborate methods of avoidance (e.g., driving her to work, protecting her from going to the cafeteria by herself, doing errands for her).

As shown in Video Illustrations 1 and 2 (see Chapter 2, "The Therapeutic Relationship: Collaborative Empiricism in Action"), Gina was able to collaborate effectively in working toward reaching her goals of 1) reducing panic attacks to one a week or less, 2) being able to go to crowded places such as the cafeteria by herself without feeling nervous or having a panic attack, 3) being able to ride elevators, and 4) driving wherever she wanted to go. Her diagnoses were panic disorder with agoraphobia and elevator phobia.

In its case conceptualization guidelines, the Academy of Cognitive Therapy recommends that clinicians take both a *cross-sectional* and a *longitudinal* view of the cognitive and behavioral factors that may be influencing symptom expression. The cross-sectional part of the formulation involves looking at current patterns of how major precipitants (e.g., large-scale stressors such as a relationship breakup, job loss, new onset of a serious medical illness) and activating situations (commonly occurring events such as arguments with one's spouse, pressures at work, being exposed to a trigger for recurring anxiety symptoms) stimulate automatic thoughts, emotions, and behaviors. The longitudinal view takes developmental events and other formative influences into account, especially as they pertain to the shaping of core beliefs or schemas.

The case formulation worksheet shown in Figure 3–2 contains a cross-sectional analysis of three typical events in Gina's current environment that are associated with maladaptive cognitions, emotions, and behavior. In her response to the first event, going to a crowded cafeteria, she has automatic thoughts such as "I'll drop my tray....I'll faint....I'll die." The emotions and physical reactions associated with these cognitions are anxiety, panic, sweating hands, and rapid breathing. Her typical behavioral response is to avoid going to the cafeteria altogether or to engage in safety behaviors (actions that diminish anxiety but prevent her from truly confronting her fears), such as going early in the morning before any crowds arrive or having a friend accompany her. The second and third examples of situations that stir up automatic thoughts and anxiety (riding in an elevator and driving to work) have similar outcomes. Her cognitions center on themes of high risk or danger and her incapacity to manage the situation (e.g., "The elevator will fall....It will be crowded, and I'll get stuck....I'll faint while I'm driving....I'll have a wreck....I'll kill somebody on the highway").

From the longitudinal perspective, Gina had early experiences (e.g., the illness and death of her grandmother; a tense and worried mother) that appeared to have contributed to the development of maladaptive core beliefs about the dangerousness of the world around her and her vulnerability to having a disaster befall her (e.g., "I'm bound to be hurt....I'm the one who will be in an accident....The world is a very dangerous place....You must always protect yourself").

Putting all of these observations together, Dr. Wright developed a working hypothesis that included these key features: 1) Gina was exhibiting the classic cognitive-behavioral features of anxiety disorders: unrealistic fears of situations, underestimates of her ability to control or manage these situations, intense emotional and autonomic arousal, and avoidance of the feared situation; 2) a developmental background of tension, wariness of danger, and illnesses and death of loved ones—and a family history of possible anxiety disorder in her mother—were likely contributors to the disorder; and 3) current situational factors (a new job and pressure to drive) may have played a role in triggering symptoms.

The treatment plan organized by Dr. Wright was directly linked to this working hypothesis. He decided to focus on modifying Gina's catastrophic automatic thoughts with Socratic questioning, examining the evidence, and thought recording. He also planned to give her training in breathing to reduce or resolve the hyperventilation she experienced in panic attacks. The most important part of the program was desensitization to the feared stimuli by developing a hierarchy for graded exposure and modeling of new behaviors to manage anxiety in feared situations. These methods are explained in detail and illustrated with videos in Chapter 5, "Working With Automatic Thoughts," and Chapter 7, "Behavioral Methods II: Reducing Anxiety and Breaking Patterns of Avoidance."

Although Dr. Wright believed that Gina's developmental experiences (e.g., her grandmother's illness and death, her sister's congenital heart disease, messages from her family about guarding against risk) set her up for having anxiety-ridden core beliefs, he opted to target most of his treatment efforts on using cognitive techniques to identify and change automatic thoughts and to implement behavioral strategies to break her pattern of avoidance. These methods are consistent with the cognitive-behavioral model for treatment of anxiety. Later in therapy, he was able to help Gina understand and modify her schemas about vulnerability to danger.

Another case shown in the video illustrations that accompany this book demonstrates how to develop a conceptualization for a person with depression. Chapter 4, "Structuring and Educating," Chapter 6, "Behavioral Methods I: Improving Energy, Completing Tasks, and Solving Problems," and Chapter 8, "Modifying Schemas," contain videos from the treatment of Ed, a middle-aged newspaper writer who became depressed after experiencing the breakup of his relationship with a girlfriend. We recommend that you wait until Chapters 4, 6, and 8 to watch the videos from Dr. Thase's treatment of Ed because they will give specific examples of how to perform the techniques described in these sections of the book. However, we briefly describe the case here as another example of a CBT case formulation. This conceptualization (Figure 3–3) should help you better understand the methods Dr. Thase chose in this example of CBT for depression.

Case Example

Ed is a 42-year-old man who has started treatment with CBT after experiencing a second episode of depression. His first bout of depression occurred about 5 years ago when he was going through a divorce. Treatment with an antidepressant and supportive therapy was helpful in reducing symptoms of depression. Nevertheless, Ed recalled that he "lost a lot of confidence" after the divorce and never returned to the state of well-being that he had achieved before having marital difficulties. He stopped taking the antidepressant after about 9 months of treatment.

Ed had been dating his girlfriend, Gwen, for about 2 years and had thought that the relationship was going fairly well. So her decision to end the relationship because it was "going nowhere" took him by surprise. During the 3 months since the breakup with Gwen, Ed had noticed a steady increase in symptoms of depression. He had very low energy, a lack of interest in his usual activities (playing tennis with friends, reading, cooking), poor sleep at night, a tendency to want to stay in bed in the morning, difficulty concentrating and organizing his efforts at work, and social isolation. His self-esteem had suffered a significant blow with the breakup, and now Ed was having many negatively charged automatic thoughts about his basic competence and his lovability. Fortunately, Ed was not having suicidal thoughts. He valued his relationship with his daughter very highly and also was proud of his job as a newspaper writer. Ed was hopeful that he would be able to benefit from treatment and learn to control his depression.

Ed's childhood years had been marked by a troubled relationship with his father. Although Ed reported that he loved his father, who was now retired and living in another state, family life had been rough. His father

Patient Name: Ed

Diagnoses/Symptoms: Major depression. Primary symptoms are loss of energy and interest, difficulty completing tasks, impaired concentration, sleeping too much, low self-esteem, and social isolation.

Formative Influences: Father had multiple job losses, was often depressed, and occasionally became verbally abusive to Ed. Family was under constant financial stress. Ed compared himself negatively to friends who seemed to "have it all," experienced academic problems during freshman year in college, and participated in athletics but always viewed himself as less capable than others.

Situational Issues: Recent breakup with girlfriend, job pressures, divorce from wife, concerns about relationship with daughter.

Biological, Genetic, and Medical Factors: Father and paternal grandmother had depression. No history of medical illnesses.

Strengths/Assets: College education; good job; history of awards in journalism; relationship with daughter; previous interest in athletics.

Treatment Goals: 1) Resume normal activity level at work and home, 2) be fully effective at work, 3) build self-esteem to a healthy level, and 4) communicate effectively with daughter.

Event 1	Event 2	Event 3
Thinking about the breakup with Gwen	Facing a deadline at work	I pick up my daughter at my ex-wife's house. I see my ex-wife briefly, and she scowls at me.
Automatic Thoughts	**Automatic Thoughts**	**Automatic Thoughts**
"What did I do wrong?" "I didn't do things right." "How could I have messed this up?" "I'll never be with somebody."	"I'm woefully behind." "I'm messing up again." "I wish I were back in bed."	"I was a failure as a husband." "I'm no good at intimate relationships." "My daughter is the only person who likes me." "What kind of jerk am I?"

Figure 3–3. Case formulation worksheet for Ed.

Emotions	Emotions	Emotions
Sad	Tense, anxious, sad	Sad, angry
Behaviors	**Behaviors**	**Behaviors**
Deflated; stay in bed in the morning and not face the world.	Irritable, worried, want to leave work, not effective in organizing assignments for the project.	Act tense and unhappy during first part of visit with daughter; avoid talking with daughter about the time she spends with her mother.

Schemas: "I'm worthless"; "I'm defective"; "If people really knew me, they would realize I'm a fraud"; "I'll end up by myself."

Working Hypothesis: Ed's divorce and the recent breakup of a relationship with a girlfriend have reinforced underlying schemas about self-worth, lovability, and competence. He has many negative automatic thoughts that are driven by these underlying schemas. His behavioral pattern of withdrawal, reduced involvement in pleasurable activities, and lack of organization at work have deepened his depression and aggravated his low self-esteem. Ed's maladaptive schemas appear to have been shaped by early negative experiences with his father (verbal abuse, father's depression and job losses), financial problems in his family, and academic difficulties in college.

Treatment Plan: 1) Behavioral interventions (activity scheduling and graded task assignments) geared at reactivation, improved ability to organize day, decreased social isolation, and improved work performance; 2) modifying negative automatic thoughts with thought records, examining the evidence, and developing rational alternatives; 3) building self-esteem and personal effectiveness by revising maladaptive schemas (identifying and listing schemas, examining the evidence, using CBT rehearsal for modified schemas); and 4) pharmacotherapy with a selective serotonin reuptake inhibitor (SSRI).

Figure 3–3. Case formulation worksheet for Ed.

had experienced a great deal of employment instability, being fired or laid off from many different jobs; his father had also had depression off and on for many years. Ed remembered his father as being a very negative man who was often irritable and was occasionally hypercritical and verbally abusive. When he was growing up, Ed preferred to spend time at his friend Kevin's house. Kevin seemed to "have it all"—a great family, money, athletic talent, and so on. However, Ed saw himself and his family as being losers.

Despite his problems at home, Ed did well in high school and had success on the track team. He continued to participate in track when he went to college, but he was never satisfied with his performance. During his freshman year in college, he had some academic problems. Nevertheless, he became very interested in journalism, began to write for the school paper, and was able to substantially improve his academic record. For the past 12 years, Ed has been a lead writer for a newspaper.

The case conceptualization shown in Figure 3–3 brings together Dr. Thase's major observations on Ed's history and cognitive-behavioral pathology to form a working hypothesis and a plan for implementing CBT. As you will note, Dr. Thase decided to add an antidepressant to the treatment program. Ed had recurrent depression, had a strong family history of this illness, and was experiencing enough symptoms to suggest that a combined approach might offer the best chance of remission. The CBT elements of the plan were directed at reversing low activity levels, the lack of interest, and social isolation in addition to helping Ed build his self-esteem and modify long-standing negative core beliefs.

The two examples of case formulations presented here demonstrate typical CBT conceptualizations for treatment of anxiety disorders and depression. In each example, the therapist brings together observations from the patient's current functioning, developmental history, and biomedical background and articulates a hypothesis consistent with the cognitive-behavioral model. The treatment plans flow directly from the working hypothesis and are rooted in specific CBT constructs for the treatment of anxiety and depression. We recommend that you begin to use the CBT case formulation worksheet now by completing Learning Exercise 3–1 and that you continue to build skills in performing conceptualizations as you gain additional experience in CBT. Chapter 11, "Building Competence in Cognitive-Behavior Therapy," includes exercises in writing out full case conceptualizations and performing self-ratings on your ability to carry out this important function.

Learning Exercise 3–1. CBT Case Formulation Worksheet

1. Use the CBT case formulation worksheet (see Appendix 1, "Worksheets and Checklists") to develop a conceptualization for a patient you are treating.

2. Try to fill out as much of the form as possible. However, if you have not performed case conceptualizations before or are inexperienced with CBT, don't worry if all of the worksheet is not completed. If possible,

identify at least one event that stimulates automatic thoughts, emotions, and a behavioral response. Also attempt to identify at least one underlying schema. If the patient hasn't reported any schemas yet, you can theorize about schemas that might be present.

3. Sketch out a preliminary working hypothesis and treatment plan based on your current knowledge of the patient and the basic CBT concepts you have already learned.

4. Continue to use the CBT case formulation worksheet as you treat additional patients with CBT.

Summary

Assessment for CBT includes all the usual tasks of performing an initial evaluation, including taking a thorough history, evaluating the patient's strengths, and performing a mental status examination. However, special attention is devoted to eliciting typical patterns of automatic thoughts, schemas, and coping behaviors and to judging the patient's suitability for CBT. Because CBT has been shown to be effective for a wide range of conditions—including major depression, anxiety disorders, and eating disorders—and can add to the effects of medication in the treatment of severe psychiatric disorders (e.g., schizophrenia and bipolar disorder), there are many indications for this treatment approach.

A broad, cognitive-behavioral-social-biological viewpoint is suggested for case formulation and treatment planning. To construct a refined and highly functional conceptualization, clinicians need to 1) perform a detailed assessment, 2) develop a cross-sectional analysis of the cognitive-behavioral elements of typical stressful situations in the patient's current life, 3) consider longitudinal (i.e., developmental) influences on the patient's core beliefs and habitual behavioral strategies, 4) formulate a working hypothesis, and 5) design a treatment plan that directs effective CBT techniques at the patient's key problems and strengths.

References

Beck AT, Freeman A: Cognitive Therapy of Personality Disorders. New York, Guilford, 1990

Beck AT, Wright FD, Newman CF, et al: Cognitive Therapy of Substance Abuse. New York, Guilford, 1993

Bryant MJ, Simons AD, Thase ME: Therapist skill and patient variables in homework compliance: controlling an uncontrolled variable in cognitive therapy outcome research. Cognit Ther Res 23:381–399, 1999

Burns DD, Rude SS, Simons AD, et al: Does learned resourcefulness predict the response to cognitive behavioral therapy for depression? Cognit Ther Res 18:277–291, 1994

Butler AC, Beck JS: Cognitive therapy outcomes: a review of meta-analyses. Journal of the Norwegian Psychological Association 37:1–9, 2000

Davanloo H: Evaluation and criteria for selection of patients for short-term dynamic psychotherapy. Psychother Psychosom 29:307–308, 1978

Dobson KS: A meta-analysis of the efficacy of cognitive therapy for depression. J Consult Clin Psychol 57:414–419, 1989

Fennell MJV, Teasdale JC: Cognitive therapy for depression: individual differences and the process of change. Cognit Ther Res 11:253–271, 1987

Frank JD: Persuasion and Healing. Baltimore, MD, Johns Hopkins University Press, 1973

Lam DH, Watkins ER, Hayward P, et al: A randomized controlled study of cognitive therapy for relapse prevention for bipolar affective disorder: outcome of the first year. Arch Gen Psychiatry 60:145–152, 2003

Linehan MM, Armstrong HE, Suarez A, et al: Cognitive-behavioral treatment of chronically parasuicidal borderline patients. Arch Gen Psychiatry 48:1060–1064, 1991

Malan DJ: The Frontiers of Brief Psychotherapy. New York, Plenum, 1973

Mercier MA, Stewart JW, Quitkin FM: A pilot sequential study of cognitive therapy and pharmacotherapy of atypical depression. J Clin Psychiatry 53:166–170, 1992

Prochaska JO, DiClemente CC: The transtheoretical approach, in Handbook of Psychotherapy Integration. Edited by Norcross JC, Goldfried MR. New York, Basic Books, 1992, pp 301–334

Rector NA, Beck AT: Cognitive behavioral therapy for schizophrenia: an empirical review. J Nerv Ment Dis 189:278–287, 2001

Rude SS: Relative benefits of assertion or cognitive self-control treatment for depression as a function of proficiency in each domain. J Consult Clin Psychol 54:390–394, 1986

Safran JD, Segal ZV: Interpersonal Process in Cognitive Therapy. New York, Basic Books, 1990

Sensky T, Turkington D, Kingdon D, et al: A randomized controlled trial of cognitive-behavioral therapy for persistent symptoms in schizophrenia resistant to medication. Arch Gen Psychiatry 57:165–172, 2000

Shaw BF, Elkin I, Yamaguchi J, et al: Therapist competence ratings in relation to clinical outcome in cognitive therapy of depression. J Consult Clin Psychol 67:837–846, 1999

Sifneos PE: Short-Term Psychotherapy and Emotional Crisis. Cambridge, MA, Harvard University Press, 1972

Thase ME: Cognitive-behavioral therapy for substance abuse disorders, in American Psychiatric Press Review of Psychiatry, Vol 16. Edited by Dickstein LJ, Riba MB, Oldham JM. Washington, DC, American Psychiatric Press, 1997, pp 45–71

Thase ME, Callan JA: The role of homework in cognitive behavior therapy of depression. Journal of Psychotherapy Integration (in press)

Whisman MA: Mediators and moderators of change in cognitive therapy of depression. Psychol Bull 114:248–265, 1993

Wright JH, Beck AT, Thase ME: Cognitive therapy, in The American Psychiatric Publishing Textbook of Clinical Psychiatry, 4th Edition. Edited by Hales RE, Yudofsky SC. Washington, DC, American Psychiatric Publishing, 2003, pp 1245–1284

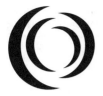

4

Structuring and Educating

To understand the value of structuring in cognitive-behavior therapy (CBT), place yourself for a moment in the position of a patient who is just starting treatment. Try to imagine what it would be like to be a person with deep depression who is overwhelmed by life stresses, who is having trouble concentrating, and who has little or no idea of how therapy will work. Add to this mix of confusion and symptomatic distress a sense of demoralization—a belief that you have expended most or all of your personal resources and have not been able to find a solution to your problems. You are feeling frightened and are not sure where to turn for help. If you were in this state of mind, what do you think you would be looking for in therapy?

Of course you would want a kind, empathic, wise, and highly skilled therapist, as we discuss in Chapter 2, "The Therapeutic Relationship: Collaborative Empiricism in Action." But you would probably also be looking for a clear direction—a hopeful and compelling path toward recovery from your symptoms. Structuring methods, beginning with goal formulation and agenda setting, can play a large role in providing a direction for change (Table 4–1). If the patient has been feeling defeated by a problem or is vexed by his inability to overcome a symptom, structuring methods can send a powerful message: *Stay focused on the key problems, and answers will follow.* Psychoeducation sends a related message of hope: *These methods can work for you.*

Table 4–1.   Structuring methods for cognitive-behavior therapy

Goal setting
Agenda setting
Performing symptom checks
Bridging sessions
Providing feedback
Pacing sessions
Assigning homework
Using therapy tools (recurrent)

Structuring and educating go hand in hand in CBT because these therapy processes complement one another in promoting learning. Effective structuring techniques enhance learning by keeping treatment well organized, efficient, and on target. Good psychoeducational interventions, such as homework exercises and using a therapy notebook, contribute important elements to the structure of CBT. The overall goals of structuring and educating are to generate hope, boost the learning process, improve the efficiency of therapy, and help the patient build effective coping skills.

During the early part of treatment, the clinician may do a large part of the work in structuring and educating. However, as CBT proceeds to its conclusion, the patient takes increasing responsibility for defining and managing problems, staying on task in working toward change, and applying the core concepts of CBT in everyday life.

Structuring CBT

Goal Setting

The process of developing treatment goals provides a great opportunity to teach the patient the value of setting specific, measurable targets for change. Typically, the first goal-setting intervention is performed toward the end of the first session, when you have assessed the patient's main problems, strengths, and resources and have started to build a collaborative empirical relationship. If you take a few moments to educate the patient about effective goal setting, the process may go more smoothly, take less time, and lead to a better result. The following case example demonstrates how to introduce goal setting in the first session.

Case Example

Janet is a 36-year-old woman who recently ended a long-term relationship with a boyfriend. She has told the therapist that the relationship was "going nowhere." Janet decided to make the change because she believed she had "wasted enough time already." Despite believing that she had made the correct decision, Janet was very depressed. She blamed herself for being "stupid to stay with him for so long" and for "putting up with a loser." Janet's self-esteem was at rock bottom. She saw herself as a person who would not find happiness in life and was doomed to be "rejected by anybody I would really want." Since the breakup 6 weeks ago, Janet had stopped exercising and socializing with friends. She was sleeping, or trying to sleep, much of the time that she was not at work. Fortunately, Janet had not been thinking of suicide. During the earlier part of the session, she had told the therapist that she knew she had to get over the breakup and put her life back together.

Therapist: We've had a good talk so far, and I think we've learned a lot about your problems and your strengths. Could we try to set some goals for treatment?

Janet: Yes. I need to stop falling apart. I've been such a wimp about this whole thing.

Therapist: I think you're putting yourself down. But let's try to come up with some goals that will give you a sense of direction—that will point your way out of this depression.

Janet: I don't know…I guess I just want to be happy again. I don't like feeling this way.

Therapist: Getting better can be an ultimate goal of treatment. But what might help the most right now is to choose some specific objectives that will tell us what we want to focus on in our therapy sessions. You might try to pick some short-term goals that we could accomplish fairly soon and some longer-range goals that will stretch us to keep working on the things that are most important to you.

Janet: Well, I want to do something with my life now besides trying to sleep it away. One goal could be to get back into my exercise routine. And I need to find something to do with my time that takes my mind off the relationship with Randy.

Therapist: Those are two good short-term goals. Could we put down on our list that you will work toward resuming regular exercise and developing positive interests or activities to help you get over the relationship?

Janet: Sure. I'd like to do both of those things.

Therapist: It also would be good to state the goals in a way that we can tell when we are making progress. What kind of markers could we set that will let us know how we are coming along?

Janet: To be exercising at least three times a week.

Therapist: How about for the interests and activities?

Janet: Well, at least going out with friends once a week and not spending so much time in bed.

Therapist: Those goals will give us a good start. Could you try to write down some other short-term goals before our next session?

Janet: OK.

Therapist: Now let's try to set some longer-term goals for us to work on. We've talked about your low self-esteem. Do you want to do anything about that problem?

Janet: Yes, I'd like to feel good about myself again. I don't want to spend the rest of my life feeling like a failure.

Therapist: Can you put the goal into specific terms? What do you want to accomplish?

Janet: To see myself as a strong person who will be fine with or without a man in my life.

The therapeutic interchange continued with the therapist giving Janet positive feedback for articulating clear goals that could help her make productive changes. Then the therapist helped Janet articulate additional goals before closing the session with homework assignments related to the overall objectives of the therapy. [The technique used here, behavioral activation, is covered in more detail in Chapter 6, "Behavioral Methods I: Improving Energy, Completing Tasks, and Solving Problems."]

Therapist: What steps could you take in this next week to make some progress toward meeting your goals? Can you pick one or two things that you could do that would make you feel better if you were able to accomplish them?

Janet: I'll go to my health club after work at least twice, and I'll call my friend Terry to see if she wants to go to a movie.

Goals should be reviewed and revised at regular intervals (at least every fourth session) throughout the treatment process. Sometimes goals set early in treatment become less important as issues or concerns are resolved or as you get to know the patient better. New goals may become apparent as therapy progresses, and adjustments in treatment methods may be needed to surmount barriers in reaching certain goals. Many cognitive-behavior therapists devise a reminder system to keep them centered on goal definition and goal attainment throughout the course of treatment. If you have a paper chart, you can include a treatment planning document that lists goals and the dates they have been reviewed. One of us (J.H.W.) uses an electronic medical record that has a first-page section for treatment goals that is displayed at each visit. You can also ask patients to record their treatment goals in a therapy notebook (see the "Psychoeducation" section later in this chapter). Some basic principles for effective goal setting in CBT are reviewed in Table 4–2.

Agenda Setting

The agenda-setting process runs parallel to goal setting and uses many of the same principles and methods. In contrast to goal setting, which is directed at the entire course of therapy, agenda setting is used to structure individual sessions. As we noted in describing goal-setting methods, patients usually need to be educated on the benefits and methods of devis-

---

Table 4–2. Tips for goal setting in cognitive-behavior therapy (CBT)

Educate the patient on goal-setting techniques.

Try to avoid sweeping, overgeneralized goals that may be difficult to define or attain. Generating goals of this type may make the patient feel worse, at least temporarily, if they seem overwhelming or unreachable.

Be specific.

Guide patients to choose goals that address their most significant concerns or problems.

Choose some short-term goals that you believe could likely be attained in the near future.

Develop some long-term goals that will require more extensive work in CBT.

Try to use terms that make goals measurable and will help you gauge progress.

---

ing a productive agenda. During the first few sessions, the therapist may need to take the lead in shaping the agenda. However, most patients quickly learn the value of an agenda and come to subsequent sessions prepared to focus on specific concerns.

Session agendas that are especially effective include some of the following features:

1. *Agenda items relate directly to the overall goals of therapy.* Session agendas should help you reach treatment goals. If you find that an agenda item is not linked to the overall goals of therapy, consider revising either the session agenda or the goal list. Perhaps the agenda item is superfluous or has limited relevance to the overall course of therapy. Alternatively, the suggested agenda item might point toward a new or reformulated goal.

2. *Agenda items are specific and measurable.* Well-defined agenda items might be, for example, "1) develop ways to cope with the boss's irritability, 2) reduce procrastination at work, and 3) check on progress with homework from last week." Vague or overly general agenda items that would require further definition or reformulation might be "1) my depression, 2) feeling tired all the time, and 3) my mother."

3. *Agenda items can be addressed during a single session, and there is a reasonable likelihood that some benefit will result.* Try to help the patient select items, or redefine items, so that progress is possible in a single session. If the item seems too large or overwhelming, take a piece of it for work in the session or restate the item in terms that are more manageable. To illustrate, an unwieldy agenda item suggested by Janet ("I don't want to feel rejected all the time") was reformulated to make

it a workable topic for a single session ("build ways to cope with feelings of rejection").
4. *Agenda items contain an achievable objective.* Instead of merely being a discussion topic (e.g., "problems with kids, my marriage, handling stress"), the agenda item includes some potential measure of change or leads the therapist and patient to work on a specific plan of action (e.g., "what to do about daughter's problems at school, argue less and have more shared activities with my husband, reduce tension at work").

Even though agendas are a mainstay of the structuring process, there can be liabilities to dogmatically following an agenda. Too much structure can be a bad thing if it stifles creativity, lends a mechanistic tone to therapy, or prevents you and the patient from following valuable leads. When agendas and other structuring tools are used to their best effect, they create conditions that allow spontaneity and creative learning to proliferate.

Achieving the right balance between structure and expressiveness has been a recurring theme in art, music, architecture, psychotherapy, and other major fields of human endeavor. For example, the success of one of the world's most famous gardens, Sissinghurst, is often attributed to the dynamic interplay between a finely wrought structure of hedges, trees, and statuary and the abundant and free-flowing plantings of colorful flowers within these borders (Brown 1990). We view the agendas and other structuring tools of CBT as promoters of the more creative aspects of therapy, in the same way that the structure of a symphony, a painting, or a garden allows the emotionally resonant part of the composition to have greater impact.

To apply this concept practically in CBT sessions, we suggest that you routinely set and follow agendas; but remember that these structures are not set in stone. Their only purpose is to help you and the patient concentrate your energies on gaining insights and learning new ways of thinking and behaving. If following an agenda item is not helpful and it is unlikely that further work with this issue on this day will bear fruit, then move on to another topic. If a new idea comes out during a session and you believe there would be significant potential in altering the agenda, then discuss your observations with the patient and collaboratively decide on whether to move in this direction. However, stick with agendas when they are working and use them to shape your efforts to help patients change.

Because agenda setting is such an important component of CBT, we have included a video illustration of this procedure. In this vignette, Dr. Spurgeon demonstrates agenda setting during a second session. At this point in therapy, the patient, Rose, is feeling somewhat overwhelmed by a number of problems, including the recent breakup of her marriage. Dr. Spurgeon starts by briefly explaining the value of agenda setting and then asking Rose to try to target some issues for work in this session. Rose responds by telling the therapist that she wants to work on her depression. Although Rose is certainly depressed and needs to find ways to relieve her symptoms, the topic she chooses, depression, is much too general to give them direction for the session. As you will see, Dr. Spurgeon helps Rose to break down this broad concern into more specific problems that they can profitably address during this visit. Although the agenda items (i.e., exploring the impact of her husband's leaving on increased depression, working on low-self esteem triggered by her child's choice to spend time with his father, and managing anxiety associated with job hunting) do not include measurable objectives, they are appropriate for this early phase of therapy and give the patient and therapist a good framework for the treatment session. Dr. Spurgeon plans to teach Rose how to develop more refined and detailed agenda items in subsequent sessions and to build her ability to organize efforts to change.

> ▶ **Video Illustration 3.** Agenda Setting:
> Dr. Spurgeon and Rose

Symptom Checks

The basic structure of CBT sessions includes several standard procedures that are performed each time the patient comes to therapy. In addition to agenda setting, most cognitive-behavior therapists include a brief symptom check or rating at the beginning of the session (J. S. Beck 1995). Typically, patients are asked to rate their level of depression, anxiety, or other mood on a scale of 0–10 points, where 10 equals the highest level of distress and 0 equals no distress. The mood rating provides a valuable estimate of progress and also adds a consistent structuring item to the therapy session.

There are several options for the symptom-check portion of the session. You can perform a mood rating, as suggested above, or do a more detailed review of current symptoms and changes since the last visit. We generally prefer to ask enough questions to obtain an accurate picture of how the patient is doing, to assess progress, and to learn about new developments. This symptom-check and brief update segment of the session usually takes only a few minutes. Another method of performing a symptom check is to administer a rating scale such as the Beck Depression Inventory (A.T. Beck et al. 1996) before each session and then review the responses when you meet the patient. Some cognitive-behavior therapists routinely set the agenda before doing the symptom check and thus include symptom assessment as a standard agenda item. Others perform the symptom check in the very beginning portion of the session as a prelude to the agenda-setting process. In the templates for session structures provided later in this chapter (see "Structuring Sessions Throughout the Course of CBT"), we use the strategy of performing a brief symptom check as the first element of the session.

Bridging Between Sessions

Although most of the structuring effort is directed at managing the flow within a single session, it is usually helpful to ask a few questions that will help the patient follow through on issues or themes from the previous meeting. Homework, one of the standard structuring elements, ties sessions together and keeps therapy focused on key issues or interventions that stream through multiple visits. However, we recommend that you go beyond checking the homework to be sure that important directions from earlier meetings are not set aside or forgotten with the press of newer initiatives. One useful way to bridge sessions is to take a few moments early in the visit to review your therapy notes and to ask the patient to review her notebook to look for follow-up items for the day's agenda.

Feedback

In some forms of psychotherapy, limited emphasis is given to providing feedback to the patient. However, cognitive-behavior therapists go out of their way to provide and request feedback to help keep the session structured, build the therapeutic relationship, give appropriate encouragement, and correct distortions in information processing. It is usually recommended that cognitive-behavior therapists stop at several points in each session to elicit feedback and check for understanding. The patient is asked questions such as the following: "How do you think the session is going so far?" "Before we go on, I want to pause a moment to see if we are both on the same track....Can you summarize the main points of what we have been working on today?" "What do you like about the therapy?" or "What suggestions do you have for things you would like for me to do differently?"

Constructive and supportive feedback is also given to the patient at frequent intervals (Table 4–3). Many times the feedback is just a phrase

---

Table 4–3. Tips for giving feedback in cognitive-behavior therapy

---

Provide feedback that helps patients stick to the agenda. You can make comments such as "I think we're getting off the subject" or "You've started to talk about a new problem; before we go in that direction, let's stop to think about how we want to use the rest of our time today."

Provide feedback that enhances the organization, productivity, and creativity of the therapy session. Spot digressions, but also take note if an unexpected breakthrough or unplanned revelation appears to hold considerable promise.

Be genuine. Offer encouragement, but don't go overboard in praising the patient.

Try to make constructive comments that identify strengths or gains and also may suggest further opportunities for change. Be careful to avoid giving feedback that may make patients think you are judging them negatively or are unhappy with their efforts in therapy.

You can summarize main points of therapy as a way of giving feedback. However, it can become tedious if you are continually summarizing the content of therapy. Giving a capsule summary once or twice a session will usually suffice.

Use feedback as a teaching tool. Be a good coach, and let patients know when they are picking up valuable insights or skills. You can use comments such as "Now we're getting somewhere" or "You really made that homework assignment pay off" to highlight areas of progress or lessons you hope they will retain.

---

or two that provides direction for the session. For example, the therapist might say, "We're making good progress today, but I think we'd get the most out of the session if we put off discussing your job until next week and focused our attention on the problem with your daughter." Of course, a statement like this would be best followed by a request for feedback from the patient: "How does this idea sound to you?" In giving feedback, there can be a fine line between providing accurate information that gives the patient appropriate encouragement and making statements that could be perceived as being either overly positive or critical. These suggestions may help you give your patients feedback that is well received and that moves the therapy ahead.

Some of the impetus for attention to the feedback process in CBT has come from the extensive studies of information processing in depression (reviewed in Wright et al. 2003; see also Clark et al. 1999). The weight of evidence from these investigations suggests that persons with depression hear less positive feedback than nondepressed control subjects and that this bias in information processing may play a role in the persistence of depressogenic cognitions (Clark et al. 1999). In addition, studies of persons with anxiety disorders have found that these conditions are associated with a rigid, maladaptive information processing style. For example, a person with agoraphobia may have been told many times by family members and friends that her fears are unfounded, but the message does not get through.

We suggest that you keep these research findings in mind when you are giving feedback to your patients. You might need to help them understand that depression or anxiety can place a filter on their perceptions and that things you or others say to them may not be heard as intended. You may also want to help your patients work on skills of giving and receiving accurate feedback. An especially useful way of doing this is by modeling effective ways of processing feedback in the therapeutic relationship.

Pacing

How can you make best use of the time in therapy sessions? When should you switch to a new agenda item? How long should you continue to work on a topic when you seem to be stalled or are having trouble making progress? How directive should you be in helping the patient stay focused on the current issue? Are you moving so fast that the patient is having trouble grasping and remembering key concepts? Would it help to go back over a topic to review what has been learned? These are the types of questions that you will need to answer to pace sessions at the maximum level of productivity while maintaining an excellent therapeutic relationship.

In our experience with supervising CBT trainees, we have found that pacing skills are hard to learn from reading about therapy. The nuances of timing therapy interventions and asking questions that effectively shape the structure of sessions are best learned through repeated practice, role-playing, receiving supervision on taped therapy sessions, and watching videos of experienced therapists.

The main strategy to keep in mind as you work on pacing CBT sessions is the effective use of a problem-oriented or goal-oriented questioning style. Nondirective or supportive therapists may simply follow the patient's lead in carrying on a therapeutic dialogue. However, if you are doing CBT, you will need to actively plan and focus the line of questioning. Based on the case formulation, you will guide the patient toward productive discussion of specific topics and will usually stick with a theme until an intervention yields results, an action plan can be developed, or a follow-up homework assignment can be arranged.

Signs that there are problems with pacing of sessions might include the following:

1. *Therapy time is used inefficiently.* You note that there are many digressions and that sessions lack clarity or sharp focus. Possible solutions include 1) increasing your attention to setting a well-tuned agenda, 2) asking for and giving more feedback, 3) reviewing overall therapy goals to see if you are staying on target to reach those goals, and 4) reviewing a taped session with a supervisor to spot and correct inefficiencies.

2. *Only one agenda item is covered when two or three other important items are neglected or given only cursory attention.* There are some occasions when a decision to spend the entire session on one agenda item is the best course to take. In this situation, other agenda items can be delayed until the next visit. However, a general pattern of not covering listed agenda items suggests that you are not thinking ahead and making strategic decisions about how to use therapy time. Try having a discussion with the patient at the beginning of the session about allocating therapy time for each agenda item. You don't have to nail the timing down to the minute, but you can try to prioritize the items and get a general idea of how much time each item should take.

3. *You have difficulty making collaborative decisions on the direction of therapy.* Pacing and timing decisions are being made only by you. The patient either has not been asked to give feedback or passively accepts all your decisions and is content to let you always be in the driver's seat. Or the patient is controlling much of the direction of the session by talking incessantly without getting or accepting feedback from you. In these types of situations, there is a problem with balance in the therapeutic relationship. The flow and pace of sessions is optimized when the relationship promotes joint decision making on a) choice of topics, b) how much time and effort are spent on a topic, and c) when to move ahead to another topic.

4. *The session ends without any sense of movement or action that could lead to progress.* Well-paced sessions are typically directed toward a change that the patient can make that will help relieve symptoms, manage a problem, or prepare him to manage a future situation. If you find that your sessions are ending without any sense of resolution or forward movement, review the case formulation, devise some strategies for change, and plan ahead to the next visit. Are you suggesting homework assignments that help the patient follow through with lessons learned in therapy sessions? If not, refine homework assignments to include an action plan for change.

5. *You give up prematurely on a topic that shows promise.* This pacing problem is commonly observed in sessions conducted by CBT trainees. Generally, the yield from a therapy session is greater when a small

number of topics are discussed in depth than when a large amount of ground is covered superficially.

6. *Your skills in phrasing questions and managing therapy transitions need further development.* Although some clinicians seem to have an abundance of native talent for asking just the right questions to make sessions flow smoothly and efficiently, most of us need to practice, watch ourselves on tape, and get good supervision before we can master interviewing techniques in CBT. Viewing taped sessions is a particularly important method of gaining skills in pacing and timing. When you observe taped sessions, try to spot areas where you could have sharpened the focus of the questioning. Stop the tape and brainstorm several different options for questions you might have asked. Also watch sessions conducted by experienced cognitive-behavior therapists to get ideas on how to ask the most effective questions and make excellent therapy transitions.

There are a number of video illustrations in the accompanying DVD that demonstrate pacing techniques in CBT. We suggest that you keep pacing and timing issues in mind as you view the brief vignettes that are included in later chapters. Sources for other videos of CBT, including sessions conducted by master therapists such as Aaron T. Beck and Christine Padesky, are provided in Appendix 2, "Cognitive-Behavior Therapy Resources."

Homework

Homework serves many purposes in CBT. The most important function of homework is building CBT skills for managing problems in real-life situations. But homework also is used to add structure to therapy by providing a routine agenda item for each therapy visit and by serving as a bridge between individual sessions. For example, if homework to complete a thought record for an anticipated stressful event (e.g., meeting with a boss, attempting to face a feared social situation, or trying to resolve a conflict with a friend) was suggested at the previous visit, this assignment would be placed on the agenda for the current session. Even if the patient does not complete the assignment or has difficulty carrying it out, there are usually benefits to discussing the homework.

When assignments work out well, review points can be made so that learning is reinforced during the session. Tie-ins to the agenda for the current visit, or ideas or issues that have been stimulated by the homework, may suggest new agenda items. When problems are encountered in completing homework, it often helps to explore the reasons why the assignment was not done or why it didn't work out as planned. Perhaps you did not explain the assignment clearly. Is it possible that you suggested homework that was seen as too difficult, too easy, or not relevant to the patient's challenges?

A strategy that usually works well is to explore any barriers that the patient experienced in carrying out the assignment. Was he feeling so overwhelmed with work that he didn't think he could take the time to do the homework? Was he afraid that coworkers, children, or others would see his homework? Was he feeling so exhausted that he couldn't get organized to start the exercise? Has there been a long pattern of procrastination? Did the word *homework* set off some negative associations from experiences in school? There can be numerous reasons why patients do not follow through with homework assignments. If you can discern the reasons why this happened, you will be in a better position to make future homework assignments a more successful experience.

We discuss homework at a number of places in this book because it is one of the most useful tools in CBT. Chapter 9, "Common Problems and Pitfalls: Learning From the Challenges of Therapy," includes a section containing detailed instructions on how to troubleshoot problems with homework completion. In addition, the wide variety of interventions for changing maladaptive cognitions and behavior (e.g., thought records, examining the evidence, activity scheduling, exposure, and response prevention) described in later chapters are used extensively as homework assignments. Although your main focus in suggesting homework may be to put a CBT method into action or to help the patient cope with a troubling situation, try to keep in mind the importance of structure in CBT and the central role of homework in providing this structure.

Structuring Sessions Throughout the Course of CBT

Some elements of session structure are maintained during all phases of CBT. However, early sessions are typically characterized by more structure than later sessions. In the beginning of therapy, patients are usually more symptomatic, may have more difficulty concentrating and remembering, are more likely to be feeling hopeless, and have not yet gained CBT skills for organizing efforts to cope with problems. By the later parts of therapy, less structure should be required because patients will have made progress in resolving symptoms, have acquired expertise in using CBT self-help methods, and be taking increased responsibility for managing their own therapy. As we have noted before, one of the goals of

Table 4–4. Session structure outline: early phase of treatment

1. Greet patient.
2. Perform a symptom check.
3. Set agenda.[a]
4. Review homework from previous session.[b]
5. Conduct cognitive-behavior therapy (CBT) work on issues from agenda.
6. Socialize to cognitive model. Teach basic CBT concepts and methods.
7. Develop new homework assignment.
8. Review key points, give and elicit feedback, and close session.

Note. Examples of CBT work in the early part of therapy include identifying mood shifts, spotting automatic thoughts, making two- or three-column thought records, identifying cognitive errors, scheduling activities, and conducting behavioral activation. There is an emphasis in the beginning phases of CBT on demonstrating and teaching the basic cognitive model. Feedback is typically given and requested several times during the visit and at the end of the session.
[a]Some therapists prefer to set the agenda before performing a symptom check.
[b]Homework may be reviewed and/or assigned at multiple points in the session.

CBT is to help patients become their own therapists by the end of treatment.

In Tables 4–4, 4–5, and 4–6, we provide templates for session structures for the early, middle, and late phases of CBT. Each session includes the common features of agenda setting, a symptom check, homework review, CBT work on problems or issues, a new homework assignment, and feedback. The amount of structure and the content of the session vary as the therapy matures to its conclusion. These templates are provided for general guidance only and are not meant to be used as a one-size-fits-all system for structuring therapy. However, we have found that these basic outlines can be customized to fit the needs and attributes of most patients and to provide structures that help reach treatment goals.

Learning Exercise 4–1. Structuring CBT

1. Enlist a fellow trainee, colleague, or supervisor to help you practice structuring methods for CBT. Use role-playing to practice setting goals and agendas at different phases of therapy.

2. Ask the helper to role-play a patient who has difficulty setting agendas. Discuss options you may have for helping the patient define productive agenda items. Then try to implement these strategies.

Table 4–5. Session structure outline: middle phase of treatment

1. Greet patient.
2. Perform a symptom check.
3. Set agenda.
4. Review homework from previous session.
5. Conduct cognitive-behavior therapy (CBT) work on issues from agenda.
6. Develop new homework assignment.
7. Review key points, give and elicit feedback, and close session.

Note. Examples of CBT work in the middle part of therapy include identifying automatic thoughts and schemas, making five-column thought records, providing graded exposure to feared stimuli, and conducting beginning- or midlevel work on changing schemas. Therapy goals should be reviewed periodically throughout the middle phase of therapy, but a review is usually not placed on the agenda for every session. The amount of structure may begin to decline gradually in the middle phase of CBT if the patient is demonstrating increased skill in organizing efforts to tackle problems.

Table 4–6. Session structure outline: late phase of treatment

1. Greet patient.
2. Perform a symptom check.
3. Set agenda.
4. Review homework from previous session.
5. Conduct cognitive-behavior therapy (CBT) work on issues from agenda.
6. Work on relapse prevention; prepare for termination of therapy.
7. Develop new homework assignment.
8. Review key points, give and elicit feedback, and close session.

Note. Examples of CBT work in the late phase of therapy include identifying and modifying schemas, making five-column thought records, developing action plans to manage problems and/or practice revised schemas, and completing exposure protocols. Therapy goals are reviewed periodically throughout the late phase of CBT, and goals for work beyond therapy are formulated. There is a focus on identifying potential triggers for relapse and using procedures such as cognitive-behavioral rehearsal to help the patient stay well after therapy ends. The amount of structure is reduced in the late phase of CBT as the patient takes progressively more responsibility for implementing CBT methods in daily life.

3. Use the role-playing exercise to practice giving and receiving feedback. Ask the helper to give you constructive criticism. Are you perceived as giving supportive, helpful, and clear feedback?

4. Rehearse giving homework assignments. Again, ask the helper to give you an honest appraisal of your skills. Does she have any suggestions for how you might improve the homework assignment?

5. Implement the structuring methods described in this chapter in work with your patients. Discuss your experiences with a supervisor or colleague.

Psychoeducation

There are three principal reasons why honing your teaching skills can help you maximize your effectiveness as a cognitive-behavior therapist. First, CBT is based on the idea that patients can learn skills for modifying cognitions, controlling moods, and making productive changes in their behavior. Your success as a therapist will rest in part on how well you teach these skills. Second, effective psychoeducation throughout the therapy process should arm patients with knowledge that will help them reduce the risk of relapse. Finally, CBT is geared toward helping patients become their own therapists. You will need to educate your patients on how to continue to use cognitive and behavioral self-help methods after the conclusion of therapy. Some methods for providing this education are outlined in Table 4–7 and are described in the subsections below.

Table 4–7. Psychoeducational methods

Providing mini-lessons
Writing out an exercise in session
Using a therapy notebook
Recommending readings
Using computer-assisted cognitive-behavior therapy

Mini-Lessons

There are occasions in therapy sessions when short explanations or illustrations of CBT theories or interventions may be used to help the patient understand concepts. A lecturing style is avoided in these mini-lessons in favor of a friendly, engaging, and interactive educational style. Socratic questions can be used to stimulate the patient to get involved in the learning process. Written diagrams or other learning aids can also enhance the educational experience. We often use a circular diagram that shows the linkage between events, thoughts, emotions, and behavior when we first explain the basic cognitive model. This technique works best if you can diagram an example from the patient's life.

Two video illustrations are provided to give you examples of psycho-educational interventions in CBT. The first vignette shows Dr. Spurgeon educating Rose on the basic cognitive-behavioral model. Earlier in this chapter, you saw Rose developing an agenda during a second session (see Video Illustration 3). One of the agenda items was to begin work on the association between Rose's marital problems and her depression. Later in this same session, Dr. Spurgeon helps Rose understand the basic CBT model for depression by diagramming her responses to waking up in the morning without her husband present (Figure 4–1). The understanding gained from this psychoeducational intervention could set the stage for efforts to help Rose modify her self-condemning cognitions and cope better with her loss. Because videos of Dr. Spurgeon and Rose are used only to demonstrate the structuring and educating procedures in this chapter, you won't see further video illustrations from this case. However, you will have the opportunity to view a number of other vignettes that show ways of implementing change.

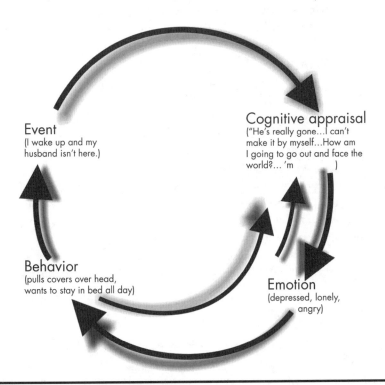

Figure 4–1. Rose's diagram of the cognitive-behavior therapy model.

▶ **Video Illustration 4.** Psychoeducation on the CBT
Model: Dr. Spurgeon and Rose

The second video illustration of psychoeducation in CBT comes from
Dr. Thase's treatment of Ed, a newspaper writer, who, like Rose, is suffering in the aftermath of the breakup of a relationship. CBT methods used
to treat Ed are also featured in Chapter 6, "Behavioral Methods I: Improving Energy, Completing Tasks, and Solving Problems," and Chapter 8,
"Modifying Schemas." A case formulation for Ed's treatment is detailed in
Chapter 3, "Assessment and Formulation." In this vignette on psychoeducation, Dr. Thase first elicits some of Ed's automatic thoughts about ending the relationship with his girlfriend ("What did I do wrong?....I don't
know what I could have done....I didn't do things right....How could
I have messed this up?"). He then explains the nature of automatic
thoughts and the connection between cognitions and depressed mood. The
vignette ends with a homework assignment to begin recording automatic
thoughts on a three-column worksheet.

▶ **Video Illustration 5.** Psychoeducation on
Automatic Thoughts: Dr. Thase and Ed

Exercise Template

A good way to educate patients on CBT methods is to write out an example of an exercise in a therapy session while explaining how the procedure works. Then the written exercise can be given to the patient as a
template for future work and a copy can be made for the chart. Seeing
the method in writing can help patients learn the concept quickly and retain it. Some possible applications of this technique include drawing a diagram of the CBT model, as shown in Video Illustration 4; writing out a
thought record (see Figure 5–2 in Chapter 5, "Working With Automatic
Thoughts"); completing an exercise in examining the evidence (see
Figure 5–3 in Chapter 5); or filling out a coping card (see Figures 5–6 and
5–7 in Chapter 5, and Table 8–5 in Chapter 8, "Modifying Schemas").

Therapy Notebook

Written exercises from therapy sessions, homework assignments, handouts, rating scales, notes on key insights, and other written or printed materials can be organized in a therapy notebook. We are strong proponents
of the use of therapy notebooks because they promote learning, can enhance follow-through with homework assignments, and can help pa-

tients remember and use CBT concepts for many years after therapy ends. For example, a man whom one of us had treated in the past called to schedule a session after a divorce. He had not been seen in the past 10 years, but he reported that he had routinely consulted his therapy notebook for assistance in using CBT to manage the stresses in his life. Although he had been troubled by the divorce, he had successfully used CBT methods to avoid slipping back into depression. After one booster session, he decided that he could continue to use self-help CBT techniques and would not need ongoing therapy.

We typically introduce the idea of a therapy notebook during the first or second session and then reinforce the value of this method throughout the course of treatment. An added bonus of therapy notebooks is that they can help structure CBT if they are consulted or augmented as a routine part of each session. Therapy notebooks are also extremely valuable for inpatient CBT applications, where the efforts of individual therapy, group treatments, homework review sessions, and other activities can be organized and enhanced with this recording method (Wright et al. 1993).

Readings

Self-help books, handouts, or other materials available in print or on the Internet are often used in CBT to educate patients and to get them involved in learning exercises outside treatment sessions. We typically recommend at least one self-help book to our patients and give them guidance on what chapters they might find helpful at different points in the therapy. For example, *Getting Your Life Back: The Complete Guide to Recovery From Depression* (Wright and Basco 2001) has two introductory chapters that help people assess symptoms and set useful goals. These chapters offer a good starting point for a person who is in the earliest stage of therapy. Chapters on automatic thoughts, core beliefs, and behavioral exercises are then recommended as therapy turns to these topics. Readings from this book about medications can be suggested when patients are receiving pharmacotherapy or are interested in learning about biological treatments for depression.

When you assign readings, try to choose materials that are appropriate for the stage of therapy; the patient's education level, cognitive capacity, and psychological sophistication; and the type of symptoms that are being experienced. In addition, materials should be selected to meet the special needs of patients. Large print may be required if patients have visual acuity problems, or audiotapes or videotapes may be needed for persons who cannot read. We keep a wide range of choices in mind when we use readings to augment CBT.

A list of recommended readings and Web sites for patients is included in Appendix 2, "Cognitive-Behavior Therapy Resources." Popular CBT self-help books include *Feeling Good* (Burns 1980), *Getting Your Life Back* (Wright and Basco 2001), and *Mind Over Mood* (Greenberger and Padesky 1996). *Coping With Depression* (A. T. Beck et al. 1995)—a brief, easy-to-read pamphlet—can be a useful educational tool for persons with severe depression. Several CBT self-help books are targeted to specific disorders or problems. *Never Good Enough* (Basco 2000) has helpful exercises for persons who struggle with perfectionism. Useful books for persons with anxiety disorders include *Mastery of Your Anxiety and Panic* (Craske and Barlow 2000) and *Stop Obsessing!* (Foa and Wilson 1991).

We suggest that you read several of the self-help books and review some of the other resources listed in Appendix 2, "Cognitive-Behavior Therapy Resources," so that you will be prepared to discuss specific educational materials with your patients. The Web sites identified in Appendix 2 can also provide valuable information on CBT. The Academy of Cognitive Therapy has an excellent Web site (http://www.academyofct.org) that has educational materials for both clinicians and consumers. The Web site of the Beck Institute (http://www.beckinstitute.org) offers suggested readings and has a CBT bookstore, and the Mindstreet Web site (http://www.mindstreet.com) supplies materials for computer-assisted CBT and also has information on the basic concepts of CBT.

Becoming an expert in providing psychoeducation requires both knowledge and practice. The next learning exercise can help you gain valuable experience in learning how to be a good teacher and coach for your patients.

Learning Exercise 4–2. Psychoeducation in CBT

1. Make a list of at least five main components of CBT for which you believe psychoeducation should be routinely provided (e.g., basic cognitive-behavioral model, the nature of automatic thoughts). What are the essential lessons you want to get across?

2. Add to this list

   a. Specific ideas for educating patients in each of the areas you have identified.

   b. Suggested readings or other educational resources for each topic.

3. Ask a colleague, fellow trainee, or supervisor to help you role-play methods for providing psychoeducation. Pay special attention to maintaining the collaborative empirical relationship and avoiding an overly didactic teaching style.

Computer-Assisted CBT

Have you thought about how computer programs might help you perform CBT? Traditional psychotherapy relies completely on the therapist to coach the patient on therapy principles, provide insights, measure progress, give feedback, and make suggestions to build CBT skills. However, there has been a growing interest in ideas for integrating computer-assisted therapy into the treatment process (Marks et al. 1998; Wright 2004). In a recent study, computer-assisted CBT with a multimedia program (*Good Days Ahead: The Multimedia Program for Cognitive Therapy;* Wright et al. 2004) was equal in effectiveness to standard CBT in treating depressive symptoms in drug-free patients, despite reducing the total amount of therapist time to 4 hours or less (Wright et al. 2005). The computer-assisted approach was more effective than standard CBT in helping patients acquire knowledge about CBT and in reducing measures of cognitive distortion.

Applications of computer technology in CBT have gone beyond the provision of psychoeducation to include a broad array of therapeutic experiences (Wright 2004). *Good Days Ahead* utilizes video, audio, and a variety of interactive exercises to help patients apply CBT principles in fighting depression and anxiety. This program also tracks the user's responses (including mood graphs, lists of automatic thoughts and schemas, action plans to cope with problems, and other data) to assist the clinician in monitoring progress and guiding the patient in use of the computer software. Two other multimedia programs for CBT have been studied in controlled trials and are being used in clinical practice. *FearFighter* (Kenwright et al. 2001), developed in the United Kingdom, is directed primarily at using behavioral methods for anxiety disorders. *Beating the Blues* (Proudfoot et al. 2003), another program from the United Kingdom, has been shown to have an additive effect to pharmacotherapy in primary care patients with depression.

One of the most interesting applications of computer technology in CBT has been the use of virtual reality to assist in exposure therapies for phobias and other anxiety disorders. Programs have been developed and tested for height phobia, fear of flying, agoraphobia, and posttraumatic stress disorder (PTSD), among other disorders (Rothbaum et al. 1995, 2000, 2001; Wiederhold and Wiederhold 2000). Virtual reality is used to simulate feared situations so that the therapist can conduct in vivo exposure therapy in the office for situations such as riding in a glass elevator or flying in an airplane. In a particularly ingenious program, *Virtual Vietnam*, Rothbaum and associates (2001) created a simulation of wartime experiences that can be used to assist treatment of veterans with PTSD.

The use of computer technology to help therapists educate and treat patients is one of the newer developments in CBT. Although some clinicians have questioned whether computer software might impair the therapeutic relationship or be perceived by the patient in a negative way, studies of computer-assisted CBT have shown excellent acceptance by patients (Colby et al. 1989; Wright 2004; Wright et al. 2002). As with any other therapy tool, you will be able to make the best use of computer programs if you make an effort to familiarize yourself with the materials and then gain experience with using them in clinical practice. Web sites that give information on computer programs for CBT are listed in Appendix 2, "Cognitive-Behavior Therapy Resources." We think that the growing use of computers in society, lack of access to empirically tested psychotherapies, and evidence for the efficiency and effectiveness of computer-assisted CBT will lead to increased use of this approach in the future.

Summary

Structuring and educating are complementary processes in CBT. Structuring can generate hope, organize the direction of therapy, keep sessions on target to meet goals, and promote learning of CBT skills. Psychoeducation is primarily directed at teaching the core concepts of CBT, but it also adds to the structure of therapy by using recurring educational methods such as therapy notebooks in each session.

Cognitive-behavior therapists add structure to treatment by setting goals and agendas, performing symptom checks, providing and receiving feedback, assigning and checking homework, and pacing sessions effectively. Another part of the therapist's role is to be a good teacher or coach. Within the framework of the Socratic method, clinicians give mini-lessons, suggest readings, and may utilize innovative teaching methods such as computer-assisted CBT. Structuring and educating methods work best when they are integrated smoothly into the therapy session and are used to support and facilitate the more expressive, emotionally charged components of therapy.

References

Basco MR: Never Good Enough: How to Use Perfectionism to Your Advantage Without Letting It Ruin Your Life. New York, Free Press, 2000

Beck AT, Greenberg RL, Beck J: Coping With Depression. Bala Cynwyd, PA, Beck Institute for Cognitive Therapy and Research, 1995

Beck AT, Steer RA, Brown GK: BDI-II, Beck Depression Inventory: Manual. San Antonio, TX, Psychological Corporation, 1996

Beck JS: Cognitive Therapy: Basics and Beyond. New York, Guilford, 1995

Brown J: Sissinghurst: Portrait of a Garden. New York, HN Abrams, 1990

Burns DD: Feeling Good: The New Mood Therapy. New York, William Morrow, 1980

Clark DA, Beck AT, Alford BA: Scientific Foundations of Cognitive Theory and Therapy of Depression. New York, Wiley, 1999

Colby KM, Gould RL, Aronson G: Some pros and cons of computer-assisted psychotherapy. J Nerv Ment Dis 177:105–108, 1989

Craske MG, Barlow DH: Mastery of Your Anxiety and Panic, 3rd Edition. San Antonio, TX, Psychological Corporation, 2000

Foa EB, Wilson R: Stop Obsessing! How to Overcome Your Obsessions and Compulsions. New York, Bantam Books, 1991

Greenberger D, Padesky CA: Mind Over Mood: Change How You Feel by Changing the Way You Think. New York, Guilford, 1996

Kenwright M, Liness S, Marks I: Reducing demands on clinicians' time by offering computer-aided self help for phobia/panic: feasibility study. Br J Psychiatry 179:456–459, 2001

Marks I, Shaw S, Parkin R: Computer-aided treatments of mental health problems. Clinical Psychology: Science and Practice 5:151–170, 1998

Proudfoot J, Goldberg D, Mann A, et al: Computerized, interactive, multimedia cognitive-behavioural therapy reduces anxiety and depression in general practice. Psychol Med 33:217–227, 2003

Rothbaum BO, Hodges LF, Kooper R, et al: Effectiveness of computer-generated (virtual reality) graded exposure in the treatment of acrophobia. Am J Psychiatry 152:626–628, 1995

Rothbaum BO, Hodges L, Smith S, et al: A controlled study of virtual reality exposure therapy for the fear of flying. J Consult Clin Psychol 60:1020–1026, 2000

Rothbaum BO, Hodges LF, Ready D, et al: Virtual reality exposure therapy for Vietnam veterans with posttraumatic stress disorder. J Clin Psychiatry 62:617–622, 2001

Wiederhold BK, Wiederhold MD: Lessons learned from 600 virtual reality sessions. Cyberpsychol Behav 3:393–400, 2000

Wright JH: Computer-assisted cognitive-behavior therapy, in Cognitive-Behavior Therapy. Edited by Wright JH. (Review of Psychiatry Series, Vol 23; Oldham JM and Riba MB, series eds). Washington, DC, American Psychiatric Publishing, 2004, pp 55–82

Wright JH, Basco MR: Getting Your Life Back: The Complete Guide to Recovery From Depression. New York, Free Press, 2001

Wright JH, Thase ME, Beck AT, et al (eds): Cognitive Therapy With Inpatients: Developing a Cognitive Milieu. New York, Guilford, 1993

Wright JH, Wright AS, Salmon P, et al: Development and initial testing of a multimedia program for computer-assisted cognitive therapy. Am J Psychother 56:76–86, 2002

Wright JH, Beck AT, Thase ME: Cognitive therapy, in The American Psychiatric Publishing Textbook of Clinical Psychiatry, 4th Edition. Edited by Hales RE, Yudofsky SC. Washington, DC, American Psychiatric Publishing, 2003, pp 1245–1284

Wright JH, Wright AS, Beck AT: Good Days Ahead: The Multimedia Program for Cognitive Therapy. Louisville, KY, Mindstreet, 2004

Wright JH, Wright AS, Albano AM, et al: Computer-assisted cognitive therapy for depression: maintaining efficacy while reducing therapist time. Am J Psychiatry 162:1158–1164, 2005

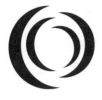

5

Working With Automatic Thoughts

Methods designed to reveal and change maladaptive automatic thoughts lie at the heart of the cognitive-behavioral approach to psychotherapy. One of the most important basic constructs of cognitive-behavior therapy (CBT) is that there are distinctive patterns of automatic thoughts in psychiatric disorders and that efforts to revise these styles of thinking can significantly reduce symptoms. Therefore, cognitive-behavior therapists often devote large portions of treatment sessions to the task of working with automatic thoughts.

There are two overlapping phases in the CBT approach to automatic thoughts. First the therapist helps the patient *identify* automatic thoughts. Then the focus shifts to learning methods to *modify* negative automatic thoughts and turn the patient's thinking in a more adaptive direction. In clinical practice, there is rarely a sharp division between these phases. Identification and change occur together as part of a progressive process of developing a rational thinking style. Commonly used methods for identifying and changing automatic thoughts are listed in Tables 5–1 and 5–2.

Items mentioned in this chapter that are available in Appendix 1, "Worksheets and Checklists," are also available as a free download in larger format on the American Psychiatric Publishing Web site: http://www.appi.org/pdf/wright.

Table 5–1. Methods for identifying automatic thoughts

Recognizing mood shifts
Psychoeducation
Guided discovery
Thought recording
Imagery exercises
Role-play exercises
Use of checklists

Table 5–2. Methods for modifying automatic thoughts

Socratic questioning
Use of thought change records
Generating rational alternatives
Identifying cognitive errors
Examining the evidence
Decatastrophizing
Reattribution
Cognitive rehearsal
Use of coping cards

Identifying Automatic Thoughts

Recognizing Mood Shifts

In the early stages of CBT, clinicians need to help patients understand the concept of automatic thoughts and assist them with recognizing some of these cognitions. We typically introduce this topic in the first session or another early session, when the patient displays a burst of automatic thoughts that drives an intense emotional response. A good rule of thumb is to regard any display of emotion as a sign that significant automatic thoughts have just occurred. Astute therapists will take advantage of these mood shifts to help uncover salient automatic thoughts and to teach patients about the basic cognitive-behavioral model.

A video illustration from Dr. Fitzgerald's treatment of Kris demonstrates how to use this technique. Kris is a line foreman at an industrial plant who is having problems at work. Depression and irritability were being triggered by job stresses, including reductions in the number of employees working on his assembly line and pressures from his bosses to meet production goals. He also was having conflicts with his wife, who criticized him about staying late at work and not participating in family activities.

In this vignette from an early session, his psychiatrist, Dr. Fitzgerald, observed a mood shift when Kris began to talk about the work situation. After noting that he appeared sad and troubled, she asked him to try to identify the automatic thoughts that were running through his mind when his mood began to change. Kris then was able to recall these thoughts: "I'm a screw-up....I can't do anything right....No matter what I do, it's not good enough....It's a stupid, dead-end job." Later in the chapter, you will see how Dr. Fitzgerald was able to help Kris modify this negative style of thinking.

> ▶ **Video Illustration 6.** A Mood Shift:
> Dr. Fitzgerald and Kris

Mood shifts are an especially useful method of uncovering automatic thoughts because they typically generate cognitions that are emotionally charged, immediate, and of high personal relevance. Beck (1989) noted that "emotion is the royal road to cognition" because thought patterns that are linked to significant emotional expression offer rich opportunities for drawing out some of the patient's most important automatic thoughts and schemas. Another reason for focusing on mood shifts is the impact of emotion on memory. Because emotional charging tends to increase a person's memory for events (Wright and Salmon 1990), therapy interventions that stimulate emotion may enhance recall and thus make it more likely that the patient will grasp and utilize the concept of automatic thoughts.

Psychoeducation

The educational methods described in Chapter 4, "Structuring and Educating," can be an important part of helping patients learn to identify automatic thoughts. We usually devote time in the beginning of therapy to brief explanations of the nature of automatic thoughts and how they influence emotion and behavior. These explanations may work best if they follow the identification of a mood shift or relate to a specific stream of thoughts that have been uncovered during a therapy session. Video Illustrations 4 and 5, shown in Chapter 4, demonstrate psychoeducation about automatic thoughts. If you haven't looked at these videos yet, we suggest that you view them now.

Guided Discovery

Guided discovery is the most frequently used technique for identifying automatic thoughts during therapy sessions. A brief sample from treatment illustrates questioning with simple guided-discovery methods.

Case Example

Anna, a 60-year-old woman with depression, had described herself as feeling disconnected from both her daughter and her husband. She was sad, lonely, and defeated. After retiring from a job as a teacher, she had hoped to have good times with her family. But now she was thinking, "No one needs me any longer....I don't know what I'll do with the rest of my life."

Therapist: You've been talking about how the problem with your daughter has been upsetting you. Can you remember an example of something that happened recently?

Anna: Yes, I tried to call her three times yesterday. I didn't hear back till 10 o'clock at night, and she seemed irritated that I had been calling her all day.

Therapist: What did she say?

Anna: Something like "Don't you know that I'm busy all day with my job and the kids? I can't drop everything to call you back right away."

Therapist: And what went through your mind when you heard her say that?

Anna: "She doesn't need me anymore....She doesn't care....I'm just a pest."

Therapist: And did you have any more thoughts—ideas that were popping through your mind at the time?

Anna: I guess I really got down on myself. I was thinking that I was pretty worthless—that no one needs me anymore. I don't know what I'll do with the rest of my life.

General methods for questioning in the guided-discovery mode are detailed in Chapter 2, "The Therapeutic Relationship: Collaborative Empiricism in Action." Some additional strategies for working with automatic thoughts are provided here. These guidelines are not absolute rules but are offered as tips for detecting automatic thoughts through guided discovery.

Guided Discovery for Automatic Thoughts: High-Yield Strategies

1. *Pursue lines of questioning that stimulate emotion.* Remember that emotions such as sadness, anxiety, or anger are signs that the topic is important to the patient. Affectively laden cognitions can serve as beacons that you are on the right track.

2. *Be specific.* Questioning for automatic thoughts almost always goes better if it is targeted on a situation that is clearly defined and memorable. Discussion of general topics often leads to reports of broadly sketched or diffuse cognitions that do not give the degree of detail needed for fully effective interventions. Examples of specific situa-

tions that might lead to discovery of important automatic thoughts are 1) "I had a job interview last Monday"; 2) "I tried to go to a party in the neighborhood, but I got so nervous that I couldn't do it"; and 3) "My girlfriend dumped me, and I'm totally miserable."

3. *Focus on recent events instead of the distant past.* Sometimes it is important to lead the questioning process toward remote happenings, especially if the patient has posttraumatic stress disorder related to longstanding issues, a personality disorder, or a chronic condition. However, questioning about recent events usually offers the advantage of accessing automatic thoughts that actually occurred in the situation and that may be more amenable to change.

4. *Stick with one line of questioning and one topic.* Try to avoid jumping around among different topics. It is more important to do a thorough job of bringing out a series of automatic thoughts in a single situation than to explore an array of cognitions about multiple situations. If patients can learn to fully identify their automatic thoughts for one problematic concern, they are more likely to be able to do this on their own for other significant issues in their lives.

5. *Dig deeper.* Patients commonly report just a few automatic thoughts or seem to get in touch with only superficial cognitions. When this happens, the therapist can ask additional questions that help the patient tell the full story. Further inquiry should be done in a sensitive manner so that the patient does not feel pushed. Questions such as the following might be used: "What other thoughts did you have in the situation?" "Let's try to stay with this a little bit longer, OK?" "Can you remember any other thoughts that might have been going through your mind?"

  If these types of simple questions don't yield results, the therapist can try to move the process along by using Socratic questions that stimulate a sense of inquiry:

Patient: When I heard that Georgette was moving to Chicago, I was crushed. She is my only real friend.
Therapist: Did you have any more thoughts about her moving?
Patient: Not really—I just know that I'll really miss her.

The therapist notes that the patient is very sad and suspects that more intense automatic thoughts are below the surface.

Therapist: I have a hunch that you might have had some other thoughts. When you heard that she was leaving, what thoughts popped into your mind about yourself? How did you see yourself right after you learned the bad news?

Patient (after a pause): That I'm not any good at making friends....I'll never have another friend like her....My life is going nowhere.

Therapist: If those types of thoughts are true, how do you see yourself ending up?

Patient: Alone....I think it's hopeless; nothing will ever change.

6. *Use your empathy skills.* Try to imagine yourself in the same situation as the patient. Get inside this person's head and think as he or she might think. By doing this with many patients, you can build your skills in understanding the cognitions that are common to a wide variety of conditions, and you will become more adept at sensing patients' key automatic thoughts.

7. *Rely on the case formulation for direction.* The case formulation, even if it is in an early stage of development, can provide invaluable help in deciding on lines of inquiry. Knowledge of precipitants and stressors will suggest important topics for discussion. Assessment of the patient's symptoms, strengths, vulnerabilities, and background history will allow the therapist to customize questions to the individual patient. One of the most useful aspects of the formulation is the differential diagnosis. If panic disorder is suspected, questions can be directed at uncovering automatic thoughts about catastrophic predictions of bodily harm or loss of control. If the patient appears to be depressed, the questioning will typically lead to themes of low self-esteem, negative views of the environment, and hopelessness. When mania or hypomania is present, the therapist will need to adjust questioning techniques to account for a tendency to externalize blame, deny personal responsibility, and have grandiose automatic thoughts. We strongly recommend that clinicians who are learning CBT acquire a good understanding of the cognitive-behavioral model for each of the major psychiatric disorders (see Chapter 3, "Assessment and Formulation," and Chapter 10, "Treating Chronic, Severe, or Complex Disorders"). This information can provide an excellent road map for using guided discovery to identify automatic thoughts.

In another vignette from the treatment of Kris, Dr. Fitzgerald asks a series of questions about the thinking that occurs when Kris is driving to his job in the morning. Even before Kris arrives at work, he is already having streams of negative automatic thoughts (e.g., "I can't do this....I'm incompetent....Other team leaders can manage, but I can't manage it"). In this example of guided discovery, Dr. Fitzgerald is able to help Kris understand that his negative automatic thoughts are contributing to his depression and his irritability on the job. They agree that these negative cognitions should be a prime target for therapy interventions.

▶ **Video Illustration 7.** Guided Discovery:
Dr. Fitzgerald and Kris

Thought Recording

Writing automatic thoughts down on paper (or on a computer) is one of the most helpful and frequently used CBT techniques. The recording process draws the patient's attention to important cognitions, provides a systematic method to practice identifying automatic thoughts, and often stimulates a sense of inquiry about the validity of the thought patterns. Just seeing thoughts written down on paper often sets off a spontaneous effort to revise or correct maladaptive cognitions. Furthermore, thought recording can be a powerful springboard for the therapist's specific interventions to modify automatic thoughts (see "Thought Change Records" later in this chapter).

Thought recording is typically introduced in the early phase of therapy in a simplified manner that helps patients learn about automatic thoughts without overloading them with too much detail. More elaborate thought recording with features such as labeling cognitive errors and generating rational alternatives (see "Thought Change Records" later in this chapter) is usually delayed until the patient gains experience and confidence in identifying automatic thoughts. One method commonly used in the opening part of therapy is to ask patients to use two or three columns to record their thinking, first in a therapy session and then as a homework assignment. A two-column thought record might include listings of events and automatic thoughts (or automatic thoughts and emotions). A three-column record could contain spaces for noting events, automatic thoughts, and emotions. Figure 5–1 shows a thought recording exercise from the treatment of Anna, the 60-year-old woman with depression described above in "Guided Discovery."

Imagery

When patients have difficulty elaborating their automatic thoughts, an imagery exercise can often yield excellent results. This technique involves helping patients relive important events in their imagination to get in touch with the thoughts and feelings that they had when the events occurred. Sometimes all that is needed is to ask patients to go back in time and to imagine themselves in the situation. However, it often helps to set the stage by using prompts or questions to rekindle their memories of events.

Event	Automatic thoughts	Emotions
My husband decided to play poker on Friday night instead of going to the movies with me.	"I'm boring. It's no wonder he wants to spend so much time with his friends. It's a wonder he hasn't left me."	Sadness, loneliness
It's Monday morning and I have nothing to do, nowhere to go.	"I'm ready to scream. I can't stand my life. I was stupid to retire."	Sadness, tension, anger
A woman at church said I was lucky to be retired and not have to deal with the students every day.	"If only she knew how miserable I am. I don't have any friends. My family doesn't care how I feel. I'm a total mess."	Anger, sadness

Figure 5–1.   Anna's three-column thought record.

Methods of using imagery to identify automatic thoughts are demonstrated by Dr. Fitzgerald in her therapy with Kris. In this vignette, Kris notes that he got very upset after coming home from work and being criticized by his wife for not attending his son's wrestling meet. At first, Kris is unable to recall the automatic thoughts that occurred in the situation. However, when Dr. Fitzgerald helps recreate the scene by asking him a series of questions that stimulate vivid imagery, Kris is able to remember thoughts such as "I'm a lousy dad….She's right…I can't even be a good parent."

▶ **Video Illustration 8.**   Imagery: Dr. Fitzgerald and Kris

The clinician's skill in explaining and facilitating imagery can make a big difference in how fully patients immerse themselves in this experience. Contrast, for example, an intervention that includes little or no preparation for imagery, followed by a rather mechanical statement (e.g., "Think back to the time you made the mistake at work, and describe what was going through your mind"), with the evocative coaching and questioning techniques used by Dr. Fitzgerald in the video illustration. Strategies for enhancing the effectiveness of imagery are listed in Table 5–3.

Role Play

Role-playing involves the therapist taking the role of a person in the patient's life—such as a boss, a spouse, a parent, or a child—and then trying to simulate an interchange that might stimulate automatic thoughts. Roles can also be reversed by having the patient play the other person and

---

Table 5–3. How to help patients use imagery

1. Explain the method.
2. Use a supportive and encouraging vocal tone. The quality of your voice and your questioning style should convey a message that the experience is safe and will be helpful.
3. Suggest that the patient try to remember what he or she was thinking in advance of the incident. "What led up to the event?" "What was going on in your mind as you approached the situation?" "How did you feel before the interaction began?"
4. Ask questions that promote recollection of the occurrence, such as "Who was there?" "How did the other people appear?" "What were the physical surroundings?" "Were there any sounds or smells that you can recall?" "What were you wearing?" "What else can you picture about the scene before anything was said?"
5. As the scene is described, use stimulating questions that intensify the image and help the patient go deeper to remember automatic thoughts.

---

the therapist play the patient. Role-playing is used less frequently than other techniques such as guided discovery and imagery because it requires a special effort to set up and implement. Also, implications for the therapeutic relationship and boundaries between patient and therapist need to be considered when deciding to use this approach. Some questions that you might ask yourself before embarking on a role-play exercise are the following:

1. *How would role-playing this particular scene with this important figure in the patient's life affect the therapeutic relationship?* For example, would the advantages of my role-playing this patient's abusive father outweigh any disadvantages of me being seen in a negative light or possibly being identified with the father? Could the role play have a favorable influence on the therapy relationship? Will the patient be able to perceive that I am being supportive and helpful by playing this role?
2. *Is the patient's reality testing strong enough to see this experience as a role play and to return to an effective working relationship after the role play is completed?* Caution should be exercised if the patient has significant characterological problems such as borderline personality disorder, has experienced severe abuse, or has psychotic features. However, experienced cognitive therapists have learned how to use role play effectively under these conditions. We recommend that beginning cognitive therapists use role play primarily with persons who have problems such as acute depression or anxiety disorders; for such patients, the role-playing experience usually will be seen as a straightforward attempt to help them understand their thinking.

3. *Would this role play tap into long-standing relationship issues, or would it be focused on a more circumscribed event?* As a general rule, it is best to orchestrate role plays early in therapy that deal with here-and-now concerns. After the patient and therapist gain experience in doing targeted role plays for specific current situations, they can use this method to explore automatic thoughts associated with emotionally loaded topics such as feeling rejected or unloved by a parent.

Despite these notes of caution, role play can be an especially useful method of revealing automatic thoughts and is typically viewed by patients as a positive demonstration of the therapist's interest and concern. Later in this chapter, we will discuss how role play can be used to modify automatic thoughts (see "Generating Rational Alternatives" later in this chapter). You will also have the opportunity to use role play as a method for learning CBT. Role play can be an excellent way for trainees to practice CBT techniques. A wide variety of therapy interactions can be simulated, stopped and started, tried in a different manner, discussed, and rehearsed. In addition, taking the patient role in training applications of this method can help clinicians get a flavor of what patients might experience in the CBT process. We suggest that you work on building your skills in role-playing and other CBT techniques for identifying cognitions by doing the following learning exercise:

> **Learning Exercise 5–1.** Identifying
> Automatic Thoughts
>
> 1. Ask another trainee in CBT, a supervisor, or a colleague to help you practice identifying automatic thoughts. Do a series of role-play exercises in which you have the opportunity to be the therapist and your helper plays a patient. Then reverse roles to expand your experiences in using the techniques.
>
> 2. Use a mood shift to draw out automatic thoughts.
>
> 3. Implement the principles of guided discovery described earlier in this chapter.[1] For example,

---

[1] See the Guided Discovery section and Chapter 2, "The Therapeutic Relationship: Collaborative Empiricism in Action."

focus on a specific situation, develop a formulation to direct the questioning, and try to dig deeper to bring out additional automatic thoughts.

4. Practice using imagery for a situation in which the "patient" is having trouble recognizing automatic thoughts. Ask a series of questions that set the scene and help evoke memories of the event.

5. Do a role play within a role play. For this part of the exercise, you will ask your helper to construct a scenario in which you will educate the "patient" on the role-play method and then use role-play methods to elicit automatic thoughts.

6. After practicing these methods with a helper, implement them with your patients.

Checklists for Automatic Thoughts

The most extensively researched checklist for automatic thoughts is Hollon and Kendall's (1980) Automatic Thoughts Questionnaire (ATQ). Although this questionnaire has been used primarily in empirical studies to measure changes in automatic thoughts associated with treatment, it can also be used in clinical settings when patients have difficulty detecting their cognitions. The ATQ has 30 items (e.g., "I'm no good"; "I can't stand this anymore"; "I can't finish anything"), which are rated for frequency of occurrence on a five-point scale from 0 ("Not at all") to 4 ("All of the time").

The computer program *Good Days Ahead: The Multimedia Program for Cognitive Therapy* (Wright et al. 2004) contains an extensive module on automatic thoughts that teaches patients how to recognize and change these cognitions. One component of the *Good Days Ahead* program is the development of customized lists of negative automatic thoughts and counterbalancing positive thoughts. Users of this program can draw cognitions from an inventory of common automatic thoughts and can also type in any other thoughts they can identify. An automatic thoughts checklist from *Good Days Ahead* is presented in Table 5–4 and is also available at http://www.appi.org/pdf/wright.

Table 5–4.   Automatic thoughts checklist

Instructions: Place a check mark beside each negative automatic thought that you have had in the past 2 weeks.

____I should be doing better in life.

____He/she doesn't understand me.

____I've let him/her down.

____I just can't enjoy things anymore.

____Why am I so weak?

____I always keep messing things up.

____My life's going nowhere.

____I can't handle it.

____I'm failing.

____It's too much for me.

____I don't have much of a future.

____Things are out of control.

____I feel like giving up.

____Something bad is sure to happen.

____There must be something wrong with me.

Source.   Adapted with permission from Wright JH, Wright AS, Beck AT: *Good Days Ahead: The Multimedia Program for Cognitive Therapy.* Louisville, KY, Mindstreet, 2004. Available at http://www.appi.org/pdf/wright.

Modifying Automatic Thoughts

Socratic Questioning

When learning to become a cognitive-behavior therapist, it is easy to fall into the trap of bypassing Socratic questioning in favor of thought recording, examining the evidence, coping cards, or other CBT methods with specific forms or procedures. However, we place Socratic questioning first in our list of techniques for changing automatic thoughts because the questioning process is the backbone of cognitive interventions to change dysfunctional thinking. Although Socratic questioning is somewhat harder to learn and to implement with skill than more structured interventions, it can pay great dividends in your effort to modify automatic thoughts. Some of the benefits of Socratic questioning are enhancement of the therapeutic relationship, stimulation of a sense of inquiry, improved understanding of important cognitions and behaviors, and promotion of the patient's active engagement in therapy.

Methods for Socratic questioning are explained in Chapter 1, "Basic Principles of Cognitive-Behavior Therapy," and Chapter 2, "The Therapeutic Relationship: Collaborative Empiricism in Action." Listed below are some key features of Socratic questioning to keep in mind as you use this method to modify automatic thoughts:

1. *Ask questions that reveal opportunities for change.* Good Socratic questions often open up possibilities for patients. Using the basic CBT model as a guide (thoughts influence emotions and behavior), try to ask questions that help patients see how changing their thinking can reduce painful emotions or improve their ability to cope.

2. *Ask questions that get results.* Socratic questions work best when they break through a rigid, maladaptive thought pattern to show patients reasonable and productive alternatives. New insights are developed, and the change in thinking is associated with a positive emotional shift (e.g., anxious or depressed mood is improved). If your Socratic questions don't seem to be producing any emotional or behavioral results, then step back, review the case formulation, and revise your strategy.

3. *Ask questions that get patients involved in the learning process.* One of the goals of Socratic questioning is to help patients become skilled in "thinking about thinking." Your questions should stimulate your patients' curiosity and encourage them to look at new perspectives. Socratic questions should serve as a model for questions that patients can start asking themselves.

4. *Pitch questions at a level that will be productive for the patient.* Considering the patient's level of cognitive functioning, symptomatic distress, and ability to concentrate, ask questions that offer enough challenge to make them think but that do not overwhelm or intimidate them. Effective Socratic questions should make patients feel better about their cognitive abilities, not stupid or dense. Ask Socratic questions that you believe the patient has a good chance of being able to answer.

5. *Avoid asking leading questions.* Socratic questions should not be used to establish the therapist as an expert (i.e., the therapist knows all the answers and leads the patient to these same conclusions) but should be a method for enhancing the patient's ability to think flexibly and creatively. Of course, you will have some idea of where Socratic questions might lead and what results you hope to achieve, but ask questions in a manner that respects patients' ability to think for themselves. Let patients do the work in answering questions whenever possible.

6. *Use multiple-choice questions sparingly.* Typically, good Socratic questions are open-ended. A large number of answers or permutations of answers are possible. Although yes-or-no questions or multiple-choice questions may be effective on some occasions, the majority of Socratic questions should leave room for a variety of responses.

Thought Change Records

Self-monitoring, a key element of CBT, is fully realized through five-column thought records and similar thought recording methods designed to help patients change automatic thoughts. The thought change record (TCR), a five-column thought record, was recommended as a high-impact procedure by Beck and colleagues (1979) in their classic book, *Cognitive Therapy of Depression*, and continues to be used heavily in CBT applications. The TCR encourages patients to 1) recognize their automatic thoughts, 2) apply many of the other methods described in this chapter (e.g., identifying cognitive errors, examining the evidence, generating rational alternatives), and 3) observe positive outcomes in their efforts to modify their thinking. We typically suggest that patients complete TCRs on a regular basis for homework and that they bring these records to therapy sessions. Sometimes patients are able to use the TCR on their own to make substantive changes in thinking. On other occasions, they may get stuck and not be able to generate rational alternatives. Regardless of the level of success in using this tool outside therapy sessions, the TCR often provides rich material for discussions in therapy and serves as a springboard for further interventions to modify automatic thoughts.

In the TCR method, two columns, "Rational thoughts" and "Outcome," are added to the three-column record typically used for identifying automatic thoughts. Patients are instructed to use the first column to write down an event or a memory of an event that stimulated automatic thoughts. The second column is used to record the automatic thoughts and the degree of belief in the thoughts at the time they occurred. Emotions are recorded in the third column.

Ratings (on a scale of 0–100), both of how much patients believe their automatic thoughts to be true and of the degree of emotion associated with the automatic thoughts, are a vital part of the thought change process. Often in the early parts of therapy, patients will rate their automatic thoughts as 100%—or close to 100%—believable. After completing the rest of the TCR and exploring ways of changing their thinking, they are usually able to produce dramatic reductions in the degree of belief in their automatic thoughts and substantial improvement in the emotional distress associated with the thoughts. Observing these changes on the TCR can be a powerful reinforcer for practicing CBT methods and using them in daily life.

Ratings of the degree of belief in automatic thoughts can also give the therapist significant leads about the malleability or resistance to change of these cognitions. Clusters of automatic thoughts that remain quite believable in the face of contradictory evidence may suggest that a deeply held schema or an ingrained behavioral pattern will need to be addressed or that more vigorous efforts to use methods such as reattribution, role play, or cognitive rehearsal will be required. Also, thoughts that persistently generate unpleasant emotions or physical tension can be targeted for more intensive CBT interventions.

The fourth column, "Rational response," is the centerpiece of the TCR. This column is used to record rational alternatives to maladaptive automatic thoughts and to rate the modified thoughts for degree of belief. Rational alternatives can be developed using a number of methods discussed in subsequent sections of this chapter. However, the TCR alone often stimulates patients to consider alternatives and to develop a more rational thinking style. Some cognitive-behavior therapists suggest that the fourth column of the TCR be used to note cognitive errors identified in the automatic thoughts, thus promoting analysis of logical errors as a way of building rational thinking. However, you can recommend that patients avoid or delay labeling cognitive errors on the TCR if you think this process would overload them or would not be beneficial at the present time.

The fifth and last column of the TCR is used to document the outcome of the patient's effort to change automatic thinking. We generally ask patients to write down the emotions from column 3 and to again rate the intensity of their feelings using a scale of 0–100. The last column can also be used to observe any changes in behavior or to record plans that have been developed for coping with the situation. In most cases, there will be positive changes noted in the outcome column. In situations where there is little or no improvement recorded in the outcome column, the therapist can use this information to identify roadblocks and to devise methods of surmounting these obstacles (see Chapter 9, "Common Problems and Pitfalls: Learning From the Challenges of Therapy").

A completed TCR from the treatment of Richard, a man with social phobia described in Chapter 1, "Basic Principles of Cognitive-Behavior Therapy," is illustrated in Figure 5–2. In this example, Richard had a flood of negative automatic thoughts as he was preparing to attend a neighborhood party. Although Richard typically avoided going to social events by either declining invitations outright or making a last-minute excuse, he was now trying to apply CBT principles to conquer his fear. Note that Richard was able to generate some rational alternatives to his automatic thoughts and that he had started to build skills for coping with anxiety (see Chapter 7, "Behavioral Methods II: Reducing Anxiety and Breaking Patterns of Avoidance," for behavioral techniques for anxiety disorders). A blank TCR is included in Appendix 1, "Worksheets and Checklists," so that you can make copies of the TCR to use in your clinical practice.

Situation	Automatic thought(s)	Emotion(s)	Rational response	Outcome
Describe	a. *Write* automatic thought(s) that preceded emotion(s).	a. *Specify* sad, anxious, angry, etc.	a. *Identify* cognitive errors.	a. *Specify and rate* subsequent emotion(s). 0%–100%.
a. Actual event leading to unpleasant emotion *or*	b. *Rate* belief in automatic thought(s), 0%–100%.	b. *Rate* degree of emotion, 1%–100%.	b. *Write* rational response to automatic thought(s).	b. *Describe* changes in behavior.
b. Stream of thoughts leading to unpleasant emotion *or*			c. *Rate* belief in rational response, 0%–100%.	
c. Unpleasant physiological sensations.				
Preparing to attend a neighborhood party	1. I won't know what to say. (90%)	Anxious (80%) Tense (70%)	1. Ignoring the evidence, magnifying. I read a lot and listen to the news on public radio. I've been practicing how to make small talk. I do have something to say. I just need to start saying it. (90%)	Anxious (40%) Tense (40%) I went to the party and stayed for over an hour. I was nervous, but I did OK.

Figure 5–2. Richard's thought change record.

Situation	Automatic thought(s)	Emotion(s)	Rational response	Outcome
	2. I'll look like a misfit. (75%)		2. Magnifying, overgeneralizing, personalizing. I'm really exaggerating here. I might look a bit nervous, but people will be more interested in their own lives than in judging how I look. I'm a competent person. (90%)	
	3. I'll clutch and want to leave right away.		3. Jumping to conclusions, catastrophizing. I will be nervous, but I need to stick it out and face my fear. I've rehearsed how to act at the party. So I don't need to leave right away or make an excuse to not attend. (80%)	

Source.   Adapted from Beck AT, Rush AJ, Shaw BF, et al: *Cognitive Therapy of Depression.* New York, Guilford, 1979, pp. 164–165. Used with permission.

Figure 5–2.   Richard's thought change record.

> **Learning Exercise 5–2.**   Using the Thought Change Record
>
> 1. Make copies of the blank TCR in Appendix 1, "Worksheets and Checklists."
> 2. Identify an event or situation from your own life that stimulated anxiety, sadness, anger, or some other unpleasant emotion.
> 3. Complete the TCR, identifying automatic thoughts, emotions, rational thoughts, and the outcome of using the thought record.
> 4. Introduce the TCR method to at least one of your patients in a therapy session. Ask this person (or persons) to complete a TCR for a homework assignment, and review the TCR in subsequent sessions.
> 5. If the patient(s) has problems implementing the TCR or is not making as much progress with this method as hoped, troubleshoot solutions for these difficulties.

Generating Rational Alternatives

In teaching patients how to develop logical thoughts, it is important to emphasize that CBT is not the "power of positive thinking." Attempts to replace negative thoughts with unrealistic positive thoughts are usually doomed to failure, especially if the patient has suffered real losses or traumas or is facing problems with a high likelihood of adverse outcomes. It may be that the patient has lost a job because of declining performance, has experienced the breakup of an important relationship, or is trying to cope with a significant physical illness. In such situations, it is unrealistic to try to gloss over the problems, ignore possible personal flaws, or minimize genuine risks. Instead, the therapist should try to help the patient to view the circumstances in the most rational way possible and then work out adaptive ways to cope.

In the book *Getting Your Life Back: The Complete Guide to Recovery From Depression* (Wright and Basco 2001), we suggested several ways that people can generate rational alternatives.[2] You might consider these options when you coach your patients on how to develop logical thoughts:

---

[2]The following list is adapted with permission of The Free Press. From Wright JH, Basco MR: *Getting Your Life Back: The Complete Guide to Recovery From Depression.* New York, Free Press, 2001. All rights reserved.

1. *Open your mind to the possibilities.* Encourage patients to be open to a full range of options. Suggest that they try to think like a scientist or a detective—someone who avoids jumping to conclusions and searches for all of the evidence. They also might imagine that they have a great coach who is building their personal strengths by helping them see positive, but accurate, alternatives. Or they can imagine what a trusted friend or family member might say about them. Each of these related strategies encourages patients to step outside their current framework of thinking to consider other viewpoints that may be more rational, adaptive, and constructive.

2. *Think like your old self.* Try to help patients get in touch with the ways that they saw themselves before they became depressed or anxious. Take advantage of the tendency for highly emotional events to be remembered in better detail than ordinary daily events. If patients can recall scenes in which they had considerable success or had a wellspring of positive feelings (e.g., graduating from school, getting married, having a child, receiving an award, being hired for a new job), they may be able to recall adaptive thoughts that are being forgotten in the crush of current problems. Ask questions such as "What alternatives would your old self see that your depressed self has ignored?" "What advice would your old self give you?"

3. *Brainstorm.* Explain the brainstorming technique. Note that artists, writers, effective businesspersons, and other creative people often try to let their imaginations run free to come up with a host of different possibilities. The first step is to list as many ideas as possible without considering whether they are practical or on target. Then the patient can sort through the possibilities to see which ones may be logical alternatives. Brainstorming can help patients break out of their tunnel vision to see options that otherwise would have gone unrecognized.

4. *Learn from others.* Often people with depression, anxiety, and other conditions turn inward and draw conclusions without the benefit of feedback or suggestions from others. Of course there are risks in asking others for their opinions. Perhaps a person who is thinking he is about to be fired, or who believes that he is unlovable, may be told that these perceptions are accurate. However, patients can be coached on ways to check out their thinking with others that will limit risks and increase the chances of success. Ask questions such as "How much can you trust this person to tell you the truth and still be supportive?" "What are the risks in asking this person for feedback?" You can also role-play possible scenarios in advance to prepare the patient to ask effective questions. Teach the patient how to frame questions that will protect her interests while still getting at the truth.

The next video illustration shows Dr. Fitzgerald helping Kris build skills for generating rational alternatives. In this example, Kris recalls an incident when he came home late from work (shown in the imagery exercise in Video Illustration 8). After his wife criticized him for missing his son's wrestling meet, Kris had a number of negative automatic thoughts ("I'm a lousy dad....I can't even do this right....He's going to hate me....I'll screw up his life"). Dr. Fitzgerald started the process of generating rational alternatives by asking Kris to tell her "the facts." However, Kris replied with more negatively toned cognitions (e.g., "I'm not there for him"). Dr. Fitzgerald then used the strategy of going back in time to ask Kris to think like his old self. This tactic worked better, as Kris began to talk about the good memories he had of camping, sporting events, and other activities experienced with his son. Then Dr. Fitzgerald asked Kris to look at the situation from the viewpoint of another person who knows him well. When he started to talk about what his friend Joe would think, Kris's thoughts about himself changed in an adaptive direction. The intervention concluded with Kris being able to generate a rational alternative to his negative automatic thoughts. Instead of putting himself down and getting more irritable and depressed, he told himself that he was "a stressed dad, but not a bad dad." This alternative stimulated him to think of ways to improve his relationship with his son.

▶ **Video Illustration 9.** Generating Rational Alternatives: Dr. Fitzgerald and Kris

Learning Exercise 5–3. Socratic Questioning and Generating Rational Alternatives

1. Practice the use of Socratic questioning and generating rational alternatives in a role-play exercise with a colleague. Try to be creative in thinking of ways to open up the "patient's" mind.

2. Next, work with one of your patients to generate rational alternatives. Focus on asking good Socratic questions. Encourage the patient to think like a scientist or a detective in looking for different ways of seeing the situation. Instruct the patient on the brainstorming technique. Your goal is to help the patient learn methods for breaking out of tunnel vision.

3. If possible, videotape or audiotape these interviews and review them with a supervisor. One of the best ways of becoming an expert in using CBT to generate rational alternatives is to see yourself in action, get feedback on your interview style, and hear suggestions on how to ask effective Socratic questions.

Identifying Cognitive Errors

Definitions and examples of commonly encountered cognitive errors are given in Chapter 1, "Basic Principles of Cognitive-Behavior Therapy." To help patients spot their cognitive errors, you will first have to educate them on the nature and types of these problems in reasoning. We have found that having the patient read about cognitive errors in a book written for the general public—such as *Getting Your Life Back* (Wright and Basco 2001), *Feeling Good* (Burns 1980), or *Mind Over Mood* (Greenberger and Padesky 1996)—or using a cognitive therapy computer program such as *Good Days Ahead* (Wright et al. 2004) is usually the most effective way to get these concepts across. You can try to explain cognitive errors in therapy sessions, but patients usually require other learning experiences, such as those noted above, before they can fully grasp these ideas. Also, providing explanations of cognitive errors in therapy sessions can be time-consuming and may divert your efforts from other important topics or agendas. Therefore, we usually briefly explain cognitive errors in a treatment session when there is an obvious example of one of these distortions in logic. Then we suggest a homework assignment to further the learning process. You can make copies of the definitions of cognitive errors from Chapter 1, "Basic Principles of Cognitive-Behavior Therapy," to use as a handout for your patients. An effort to teach a patient to spot cognitive errors is illustrated in the following case:

Case Example

Max, a 30-year-old man with bipolar disorder, reported a flare of intense irritability and anger during an argument with his girlfriend. His girlfriend, Rita, had called Max to tell him she was held up at work and would be about an hour late for a date to go out for dinner. They had a reservation for 7 P.M., but Rita didn't arrive at his house until almost 9 o'clock. By that time Max was in quite a fury. He reported that he "screamed at her for 30 minutes and then went to a bar without her."

In the therapy session, the clinician noted that Max had a number of maladaptive automatic thoughts that were laced with cognitive errors.

Therapist: Can you think back over the situation to tell me the automatic thoughts that were going through your mind? Try to speak the thoughts out loud now so that we can understand why you got so upset.

Max: She only cares about herself and her big-time job. She doesn't think about me at all. This relationship is going nowhere. She makes me look like a jerk!

Therapist: You told me that you felt guilty this morning and believe that you overreacted to her being late. You also said that you love her and want to make the relationship work. I think it might help to look at what you were thinking in the situation. It sounds like you took an extreme view of her behavior.

Max: Yes, I guess I was really wound up tight. Sometimes I get that way and go way overboard.

Therapist: One of the things that seemed to be happening was that you were thinking in extremes. Sometimes we call this "all-or-nothing" or "absolute" thinking. For example, your automatic thought "She doesn't care about me at all" is very absolute and gives no room for you to consider any other information about how she treats you. How did thinking like this make you feel and act?

Max: I got into a rage and said some really hurtful things to her. If I keep doing this, I'll ruin the relationship.

The therapist then explained the concept of cognitive errors and how spotting these distortions could help Max better manage his emotions and behavior.

Therapist: So, I've told you about these things we call cognitive errors. Would you be willing to read something about them before the next session? You could also try to identify some of these cognitive errors on your thought records.

Max: Sure. I think that's a good idea.

There can be multiple opportunities for helping patients learn how to spot cognitive errors and reduce the frequency and intensity of these distortions in logic. As mentioned above in the "Thought Recording" section, a TCR can be used to identify cognitive errors in specific automatic thoughts (see Figure 5–2). Cognitive errors can also be recognized in other interventions such as examining the evidence and decatastrophizing. For many patients, spotting and labeling cognitive errors is one of the more challenging parts of building cognitive therapy skills. These thinking errors have been repeated over and over for many years and have become an automatic part of information processing. Therefore, the therapist may need to repetitively draw the patient's attention to this phenomenon and suggest multiple ways to practice thinking in a more balanced and logical manner.

Sometimes patients can get confused in their effort to identify cognitive errors. The definitions of the various errors can be difficult to understand, and there can be considerable overlap between the different types of errors in reasoning. It is a good idea to explain in advance that it might take some time to gain experience in spotting cognitive errors. We tell patients that it's not important to label the errors exactly each time (e.g., to discriminate between ignoring the evidence and overgeneralizing) or to recognize all of the cognitive errors that might be involved in an automatic thought (many automatic thoughts include more than one type of cognitive error). We try to convey the message that they shouldn't worry about getting this part of CBT exactly right. Recognizing *any* cognitive errors can help them think more logically and cope better with their problems.

Examining the Evidence

The strategy of examining the evidence can be a powerful method for helping patients modify automatic thoughts. This technique involves listing evidence for and against the validity of an automatic thought or other cognition, evaluating this evidence, and then working on changing the thought to be consistent with the newfound evidence. There are two video illustrations of using examining the evidence to change automatic thoughts.

In the first example, Dr. Fitzgerald shows Kris how to check out the validity of his thinking about an upcoming visit from corporate executives to his industrial plant. For homework, Kris had partially completed a TCR about this anticipated event. Although he had been able to identify many automatic thoughts (e.g., "They are going to yell at me....I'm going to lose my job....I can't do anything right....I'm a loser"), he had been unable to generate ideas for the "Rational response" column of the TCR. To help Kris do this, Dr. Fitzgerald asked him to pick two of the negative automatic thoughts to use as exercises for examining the evidence. The entries from Kris's first worksheet are shown in Figure 5–3.

> ▶ **Video Illustration 10.** Examining the Evidence:
> Dr. Fitzgerald and Kris

The second video illustration shows Dr. Wright working with Gina to test the validity of her automatic thoughts about the likelihood of embarrassing herself in the cafeteria. This vignette was shown earlier in Chapter 2, "The Therapeutic Relationship: Collaborative Empiricism in Action," as an example of a collaborative empirical therapeutic relationship. We

Automatic thought: I'm going to lose my job.

Evidence for automatic thought:	Evidence against automatic thought:
1. Productivity on my line has decreased.	1. The plant is already low on employees; they won't be in a hurry to let people go.
2. I received a reprimand.	2. I've been there 10 years and have a good track record.
3. We haven't reached our goal.	3. We aren't missing production goals by much.
	4. The company doesn't have a history of firing people on a whim.
	5. No one has said anything about me losing my job.

Cognitive errors: Ignoring the evidence—I've only had one bad mark in 10 years.

Alternative thoughts: It's unlikely that I'll lose my job. They aren't coming to fire me. They are just trying to see how to improve production.

Source. Modified from Wright et al. 2004.

Figure 5–3. Examining-the-evidence worksheet.

suggest that you view this video again, with your attention focused now on learning ways to implement the technique of examining the evidence. Dr. Wright demonstrates an intervention in examining the evidence that did not include a written worksheet. Examining the evidence can be performed quickly as part of a series of therapy interventions as in this example, or can be done in a more detailed manner with worksheets as shown in Dr. Fitzgerald's treatment of Kris. Generally, we recommend that examining the evidence be implemented in its full version with listing of written evidence at least once in the early part of therapy to teach patients how to use this valuable method. Exercises in examining the evidence also make excellent homework assignments. A copy of the blank worksheet is provided in Appendix 1, "Worksheets and Checklists."

> ▌ **Video Illustration 2.** Modifying Automatic Thoughts: Dr. Wright and Gina

Decatastrophizing

Catastrophic predictions about the future are very common in persons with depression and anxiety. These predictions are frequently influenced by the cognitive distortions observed in these disorders, but sometimes the fears are on target. Thus the decatastrophizing procedure does not always attempt to negate the catastrophic fear. Instead, the therapist may elect to help the patient work on ways to cope with a feared situation in case it does come true.

Case Example

Terry, a 52-year-old depressed man who was in his second marriage, expressed great anxiety about the possibility that his wife would leave him. Because the relationship did appear shaky, his therapist decided to use the *worst-case scenario* technique to help him decatastrophize and better manage the situation.

Terry: I think she is at the end of her rope with me. I couldn't survive another rejection.
Therapist: I can tell that you are very worried and upset. What do you think the chances are of your staying together?
Terry: About 50–50.
Therapist: Because you are predicting a high likelihood of a breakup, it might help to think ahead to what would happen if she did file for divorce. What is the worst outcome that you could imagine?
Terry: I'd be destroyed...a two-time loser with no future. She's everything to me.
Therapist: I know that it would be very tough if your marriage did end in divorce, but let's take a look at how you could cope. We can start with checking out your predictions. You said that you would be destroyed. Can we look at the evidence to see if that would be true?
Terry: I suppose I wouldn't be totally destroyed.
Therapist: What parts of you or your life wouldn't be destroyed?
Terry: My kids would still love me. And my brothers and sisters wouldn't give up on me. In fact, some of them think that I'd be better off ending the marriage.
Therapist: Any other parts of your life that would still be OK?
Terry: My job, as long as I don't get too depressed to do it. I can keep playing tennis with my friends. You know that tennis is a big outlet for me.

The therapist proceeded with questions to help Terry modify his absolutistic, catastrophic thoughts. By the end of this interchange, Terry had developed a different view of his reactions to a possible divorce.

Therapist: Before we go on, can you sum up what we've learned about how you might react if you did have to face a divorce?
Terry: It would be a big blow, and I don't want it to happen. But I'd try to look at all of the things I do have instead of thinking only about what I'm losing. I still have my health and the rest of my family. I have a good job and some close friends. She's been a big part of

my life, but she isn't everything. Life would go on. Maybe I'd be better off in the long run, like my brother tells me.

The therapist then suggested that they work on a coping plan to be used in case a divorce should actually occur. [See the "Coping Cards" section later in this chapter for more information.]

Decatastrophizing also is a valuable technique for helping individuals with anxiety disorders. For example, persons with social phobia commonly have fears that they will be exposed as anxious or socially incompetent and that this revelation will be too painful to bear. You can try the following types of questions to reduce catastrophic predictions in social phobia: "What is the worst thing that could happen if you went to the party?" "What would be terrible about not having much to say?" "Could you tolerate this for at least 15 minutes?" "How does feeling anxious at a party compare with other terrible things, like having a serious illness or losing a job?" The thrust of such questions is to help patients see that their predictions of dire consequences and inability to cope are inaccurate.

The decatastrophizing technique also helps patients build confidence that they can manage feared situations. The video illustration of Dr. Wright helping Gina with her fears of eating in a cafeteria (see Video Illustration 2) shows a combination of examining the evidence and decatastrophizing methods geared toward helping Gina gain skills in confronting the situation.

Reattribution

In Chapter 1, "Basic Principles of Cognitive-Behavior Therapy," we describe the findings of studies on attributional biases in depression. Attributions are the meanings people assign to events in their lives. To refresh your memory, we briefly summarize the three dimensions of distorted attributions:

1. *Internal versus external.* Depressed persons tend to internalize blame or responsibility for negative outcomes, whereas nondepressed persons make balanced or external attributions.
2. *General versus specific.* In depression, attributions are more likely to be sweeping and global than isolated to a specific flaw, insult, or problem. An example of a generalized attribution is "That fender bender was the last straw; everything in my life is going downhill."
3. *Invariant versus variable.* Depressed persons make attributions that are invariant and predict little or no chance of change—for example, "I will never find love again." In contrast, nondepressed persons are more likely to think "This too will pass."

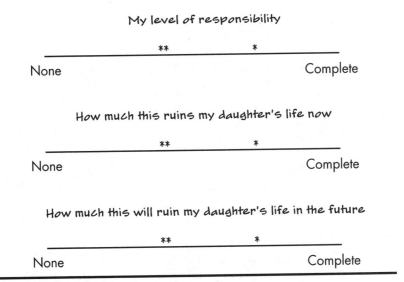

Figure 5–4. Sandy's attribution scales.
*What I think today.
**A healthy view of the situation.

A variety of different methods can help patients make healthier attributions to significant events in their lives. Any of the other techniques described in this chapter can be employed, such as Socratic questioning, TCRs, or examining the evidence. However, we typically initiate reattribution by briefly explaining the concept and then drawing a graphic on a piece of paper to demonstrate the dimensions of attributions (Figure 5–4). Then we ask questions that prompt the patient to explore and possibly change his or her attributional style.

Case Example

Sandy, a 54-year-old woman, was having trouble coping with the revelation that her married daughter, Maryruth, was having an affair. She blamed herself excessively, believed that her daughter was ruining her entire life, and thought that Maryruth's future was very dim. The therapist began with questions targeted at correcting Sandy's internalized attributions. [The diagram in Figure 5–4 was used to record Sandy's answers.]

Therapist: How much do you blame yourself for your daughter's problems now?
Sandy: A lot—probably about 80%. I should never have gone along with her idea to go to that college. She went wild up there, and she hasn't been herself since. I knew it was a bad idea for her to marry Jim. I should have told her what I thought about him. They don't have anything in common.

Therapist: We'll check out all of this blame you are putting on yourself later. But for now, can you just make a mark on the graph to show how much you think you are responsible for the problem?

Sandy places a mark at about the 90% level.

Therapist: OK, now let's try to think about what a healthy level of blame would be. Where would you like to be on the graph?

Sandy: I know I get down on myself too much. But I think I should still try to help and should take *some* of the responsibility. Probably 25% is about right.

Sandy places a mark at about the 25% level.

Although the therapist believed that Sandy was still taking too much blame for the situation, she didn't press the issue at that time. They proceeded to make graphs for the other dimensions of attributions [see Figure 5–4] and then began to discuss ways to move attributions in the desired direction.

One of the techniques that can be used to modify attributions is to ask the patient to brainstorm about a variety of possible contributors to negative outcomes. Because patients often have tunnel vision that is focused on their own faults, it can help to ask questions that prompt them to think of different perspectives—for example, "How about other people who could have influenced the situation: the in-laws? his buddies?" "What about the role of luck or fate?" "Could genetics be involved?" After going through a series of these types of questions, we sometimes use a pie graph to help patients take a multidimensional view of the situation. Figure 5–5 shows a pie graph that Sandy constructed for her attributions about blame for her daughter's problems.

> **Learning Exercise 5–4.** Examining the Evidence, Decatastrophizing, and Reattribution
>
> 1. Again, ask a colleague to help you learn CBT procedures by doing role-play exercises. Ask your helper to role-play a situation in which examining the evidence, decatastrophizing, or reattribution for changing automatic thoughts might be used.
>
> 2. Then sequentially try out each of the techniques.
>
> 3. When you examine the evidence, use a worksheet (see Appendix 1, "Worksheets and

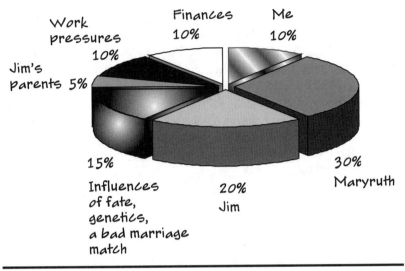

Figure 5–5. Sandy's pie graph: the positive effects of reattribution.

Checklists") and write out evidence for and against the automatic thought. Then try to spot cognitive errors (if any) in the "evidence for" column. Now help the "patient" revise and record a modified thought.

4. When you practice decatastrophizing, focus on correcting distorted predictions. But also work on preparing the "patient" to cope with possible adverse outcomes.

5. Next choose an automatic thought that might respond to a reattribution intervention. Explain attributional biases, and then use a graphic (as in Figure 5–4) and/or a pie graph (as in Figure 5–5) to help the "patient" make healthier attributions.

6. The last step in this learning exercise is to implement all three procedures with actual patients and to discuss your efforts with a supervisor.

Cognitive Rehearsal

When you are facing an important meeting or task, do you ever think through in advance what you are going to say? Do you rehearse your thoughts and behaviors so that you will have a greater chance of success? We certainly use this strategy in our own lives, and we have found that it can help patients take the lessons of therapy into real-world situations.

When we explain this technique to patients, we often use the example of top athletes, such as downhill skiers, who can visualize the challenges of a competitive situation and prepare their minds for the course ahead. A skier might use imagery to think about how she would react in a variety of situations. How would she compensate if she hit a patch of ice or a strong wind began to blow? The skier would also probably coach herself on keeping a positive mind-set to calm her anxieties and focus on competing in the race.

Cognitive rehearsal is usually introduced in a therapy session after the patient has already done some groundwork with other methods to change automatic thoughts. These earlier experiences prepare the patient to "put it all together" in orchestrating an adaptive response to a potentially stressful situation. One way of doing cognitive rehearsal is to ask the patient to take these steps: 1) think through a situation in advance; 2) identify possible automatic thoughts and behavior; 3) modify the automatic thoughts by writing out a TCR or doing another CBT intervention; 4) rehearse the more adaptive way of thinking and behaving in your mind; and then 5) implement the new strategy.

Of course, it often helps to coach patients on methods that will help them increase the chances of achieving their goals. They can be asked Socratic questions to help them see different options, mini-didactic interventions can be used to teach them skills, and experiments can be tried to test out possible solutions. However, often the most useful technique is rehearsing in a therapy session before trying out the new plan in vivo. Dr. Fitzgerald used this method with Kris to help him prepare for an upcoming visit from corporate executives.

> ▶ **Video Illustration 11.** Cognitive Rehearsal:
> Dr. Fitzgerald and Kris

Coping Cards

The use of coping cards can be a productive way to help patients practice key CBT interventions learned in therapy sessions. Either index cards (3×5 inches) or smaller cards (business-card size) can be utilized to write

---

Table 5–5. Tips for developing coping cards

1. Choose a situation that is important to the patient.
2. Plan therapy interventions with the goal of producing coping cards.
3. Assess the patient's readiness to implement strategies with a coping card. Don't try to do too much too soon. Start with a manageable task. Delay tackling overwhelming concerns or issues until the patient is prepared to meet these challenges.
4. Be specific in defining the situation and the steps to be taken to manage the problem.
5. Boil the instructions down to their essence. Highly memorable instructions are more likely to stick.
6. Be practical. Suggest strategies that have a high likelihood of success.
7. Advocate frequent use of the coping card in real-life situations.

---

down instructions that patients would like to give themselves to help them cope with significant issues or situations. When used to best effect, coping cards identify a specific situation or problem and then succinctly detail a coping strategy with a few bullet points that capture the fundamentals of the plan. Table 5–5 presents some tips for helping patients write coping cards that work.

In Video Illustration 11, Dr. Fitzgerald helps Kris record the ideas from a cognitive rehearsal exercise on a coping card. Kris wrote down these adaptive cognitions on a coping card and planned to keep the card in his wallet so that he could review it frequently before the corporate executives visited his industrial plant (Figure 5–6).

Another example of a coping card comes from the treatment of Max, the man with bipolar disorder who reported intense anger in his relationship with his girlfriend (Figure 5–7). Additional interventions described in the chapters on behavioral methods might be added later to help him deal more effectively with his anger, but Max has made a good start.

Learning Exercise 5–5. Cognitive Rehearsal and Coping Cards

1. Identify a situation in your own life for which advance rehearsal might help you be more effective or assured. Now go through the situation in your mind, identifying possible automatic thoughts, emotions, rational thoughts, and adaptive behaviors. Next, practice thinking and acting in the most adaptive way you can imagine.

Situation: Corporate executives are coming to survey our production problems.

Coping strategies:

Remind myself that

    We are very close to reaching our production goals.

    Other work groups at my plant are worse off than we are.

    They are not really looking at me. The pressure will be on my bosses.

    They're only going to ask a question or two. They're not going to interrogate me.

Figure 5–6.   Kris's coping card.

Situation: My girlfriend comes in late or does something else that makes me think she doesn't care.

Coping strategies:

Spot my extreme thinking, especially when I use absolute words like <u>never</u> or <u>always</u>.

Stand back from the situation and check my thinking before I start yelling or screaming.

Think of the positive parts of our relationship—I think she does love me.

We've been together for 4 years, and I want to make it work.

Take a "time-out" if I start getting into a rage. Tell her that I need to take a break to calm down. Take a brief walk or go to another room.

Figure 5–7.   Max's coping card.

2. Distill the efforts of your cognitive rehearsal exercise into a coping card. Follow the tips for writing coping cards in Table 5–5. Write out specific bullet points that will coach you on the best way to handle the situation.

3. Practice cognitive rehearsal with at least one of your patients. Choose a situation that you believe the patient could manage better if it were thought through in advance. Also, try to pick rehearsal opportunities that might reduce the risk for symptom worsening or relapse. Examples might include going back to work, getting bad news about the health of a relative, or being criticized by a significant other.

4. Write out a least three coping cards with your patients. Promote use of the cards by asking patients to implement the coping strategies as homework assignments.

Summary

CBT focuses on identifying and changing automatic thoughts because these cognitions have a strong influence on emotions and behavior. During the early phase of working with automatic thoughts, therapists teach patients about this stream of private, often unchecked cognitions and help them tune in to this internal dialogue. Guided discovery is the most important method used to uncover automatic thoughts, but many other techniques are available. Recognizing a mood shift is a powerful way of showing patients the impact of automatic thinking on their feelings. Other valuable methods for eliciting automatic thoughts include thought recording, imagery, role play, and the use of checklists.

After the patient learns to identify automatic thoughts, therapeutic efforts can shift to the use of interventions for modifying these cognitions. Effective Socratic questioning is the cornerstone of the change process. Thought change records are also used extensively in CBT to help patients develop a more logical and adaptive thinking style. Therapists can draw from a variety of other useful techniques—such as examining the evidence, decatastrophizing, reattribution, cognitive rehearsal, and coping cards—to revise automatic thoughts. As CBT moves from early to later phases, patients gain skills in modifying automatic thoughts that they can use on their own to reduce symptoms, cope better with life stresses, and decrease the chance of relapse.

References

Beck AT: Cognitive therapy and research: a 25-year retrospective. Paper presented at the World Congress of Cognitive Therapy, Oxford, England, June 28–July 2, 1989

Beck AT, Rush AJ, Shaw BF, et al: Cognitive Therapy of Depression. New York, Guilford, 1979

Burns DD: Feeling Good: The New Mood Therapy. New York, William Morrow, 1980

Greenberger D, Padesky CA: Mind Over Mood: Change How You Feel by Changing the Way You Think. New York, Guilford, 1996

Hollon SD, Kendall PC: Cognitive self-statements in depression: development of an automatic thoughts questionnaire. Cognit Ther Res 4:383–395, 1980

Wright JH, Basco MR: Getting Your Life Back: The Complete Guide to Recovery From Depression. New York, Free Press, 2001

Wright JH, Salmon P: Learning and memory in depression, in Depression: New Directions in Research, Theory, and Practice. Edited by McCann D, Endler NS. Toronto, ON, Wall & Thompson, 1990, pp 211–236

Wright JH, Wright AS, Beck AT: Good Days Ahead: The Multimedia Program for Cognitive Therapy. Louisville, KY, Mindstreet, 2004

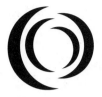

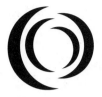 **6**

Behavioral Methods I

Improving Energy, Completing Tasks, and Solving Problems

Low energy, decreased capacity for enjoyment of activities, and difficulty completing tasks or solving problems are common complaints of people with depression. Although cutting back on activity levels may seem logical or necessary to the person who is experiencing depression, this action often results in an aggravation of symptoms. A vicious cycle can ensue in which reduced involvement in stimulating activities or in productive actions to manage problems is followed by further lack of interest, increased helplessness, or lower self-esteem. The individual may eventually conclude that he is incapable of experiencing pleasure, completing tasks, or solving problems. Patients with the deepest cases of depression may become abjectly hopeless and give up on any attempts to change.

Cognitive-behavioral methods for treating depression and other psychiatric disorders include specific interventions designed to reverse patterns of diminishing activity levels, energy depletion, worsening anhedonia, and reduced abilities to complete tasks or solve problems. In this chapter, we discuss and illustrate some of the most useful behavioral interventions for helping people with these types of difficulties. Although the techniques described here are most often used in treatment of depression, they also can be applied successfully in cognitive-behavior therapy (CBT) for other conditions, such as anxiety disorders, eating disorders, and personality disorders (see Chapter 10, "Treating Chronic, Severe, or Complex Disorders").

When you implement behavioral procedures, it is important to remember the principle that positive behavioral changes are likely to be associated with improved self-esteem or more adaptive attitudes. Likewise, modifications in negative automatic thoughts or schemas can help promote adaptive behavior. Thus, behavioral methods are used in concert with cognitive techniques as an overall strategy for reaching treatment goals. The examples in this chapter illustrate how behavioral and cognitive interventions often augment each other and how therapists can blend these techniques in clinical practice.

Behavioral Activation

We use the term *behavioral activation* to describe a simple procedure that engages the patient in a process of change and stimulates a sense of positive movement and hope. The therapist helps the patient to choose one or two actions that could make a difference in how he feels and then assists with working out a brief plan to carry out the activity. Behavioral activation is typically used in the first session or in other early sessions before more detailed behavioral analyses or interventions can be performed (e.g., activity schedules, graded task assignments). However, we have also found that this technique can be applied at other stages of therapy when an uncomplicated, targeted behavioral action can be used with benefit. The following example of behavioral activation demonstrates how this method can be used to rapidly engage patients in productive activities very early in therapy.

Case Example

During his first session, Jeremy, a 37-year-old single man, described the evolution of his depression, which had begun after he had had to close his small business about 6 months previously. His self-esteem had been so battered by the experience that he was ashamed to see his family and friends. He spent most of each day in his apartment watching television or reading. Instead of cooking or going out to dinner with friends, he sat at home eating frozen dinners or junk food. Since Jeremy stopped exercising at a local gym, he had gained more than 20 pounds. He saw himself as a "failure" or a "reject," and his behavior was consistent with these beliefs. Toward the end of the first session, the therapist used behavioral activation to help Jeremy start reducing symptoms of depression.

Jeremy: I feel like I'm wasting my life. I'm not working. I stay to myself all the time. I don't do anything interesting or fun. I'm going nowhere fast.

Therapist: What ideas have you had about things you might do to change the situation?

Jeremy: I don't know. (*Pauses.*) Well, I guess I need to get out of this rut. But I don't know where to start. After the business failed, I sort of gave up.

Therapist: I've been wondering whether there might be one thing you could do right now that would make you feel better. Maybe there is a change that you could make that wouldn't involve tackling the whole problem but would still get you going again. What action could you take in the next couple days that would begin to make a difference?

Jeremy (after pausing to think): I could call my old friend Vince and ask if he wants to go out and shoot some pool or go to the movies. We always had a good time together. I haven't gone out with any of my friends in over 2 months.

Therapist: That's a good idea. From what you told me, it sounds like being alone all the time has been making you feel worse. Is there one more thing you could do in the next week that would help you begin to break out of the rut?

Jeremy: Yes, when I was telling you about eating all that fast food, I was thinking about getting back into cooking. I used to enjoy cooking—even when I ate by myself. I know how to make good food that won't pile the calories on.

Therapist: Another good idea. So let's get specific with your plan. We decided to schedule another session next week. What will you do before we meet again?

Jeremy: I'll call Vince and arrange to do something this weekend. If Vince can't do it, I'll call another friend.

Therapist: Great. What about your idea to start cooking again? What would you like to cook? What will you plan to do?

Jeremy: I'm not ready to entertain anyone, but I can look through my recipes and go shopping for the stuff to make a couple good meals for myself.

Because Jeremy was severely depressed and was having difficulty engaging in any activities that gave him a sense of well-being or pleasure, the therapist was careful to avoid suggesting a behavioral activation plan that would be too challenging or would be unlikely to be accomplished. In this case, the patient chose some actions that were within his reach, had a good chance of stimulating an increased sense of pleasure, and were unlikely to lead to further experiences of failure. If the patient had suggested behaviors that would have been especially difficult to execute or would have presented high risks for negative outcomes, the therapist would have helped him choose some other options with a better chance of success.

When patients come to their first session, they are usually interested in making changes. They want to start moving in a positive direction, and they are looking for guidance for steps they can begin to take. Therefore, when the therapist suggests taking an immediate behavioral action (even if it is rudimentary), this request is usually greeted by patients as a sign that they will be able to work together with the therapist on making bigger gains and on solving larger problems. Behavioral activation isn't a fancy or complicated technique, but it can help patients start to break out of patterns of withdrawal or inactivity, show them that progress can be made, and stimulate hope for recovery. This type of intervention may also be used to good effect in later stages of therapy or in the maintenance phase of treatment of chronic conditions.

Case Example

Georgine, a woman with bipolar disorder, was being seen by a psychiatrist with expertise in CBT for 20-minute sessions about once a month. Although her psychiatrist had recently added lamotrigine to her previous pharmacotherapy regimen of lithium and risperidone, Georgine had been experiencing moderate depressive symptoms for over 2 months.

When Georgine reported that she had stopped singing in her church choir, had dropped out of adult education classes, and was spending much more time sleeping during the day than usual, her psychiatrist became worried that the reduced activity would become part of a downward spiral that would further aggravate her depression. Instead of using the more detailed techniques of activity scheduling and graded task assignments described later in the chapter, he elected to try a simple behavioral activation exercise.

Therapist: I'm concerned that stopping some of your favorite activities—like singing in the choir and taking classes—might end up making you feel worse. What do you think?

Georgine: I guess you're right. But when I'm depressed, I just don't have the energy to do all that stuff. I feel like curling up at home and not facing the world.

Therapist: And what happens when you spend most of the day in bed or on your couch?

Georgine: It feels better at first, but then I start thinking that I don't matter or that no one cares.

Therapist: Can you think of one thing you could do in this next week to spend less time on the couch? If you're not feeling up to rejoining the choir, I'll bet there is something else you could do that might be worth considering.

Georgine: I get your point. Dropping out of everything isn't a very good idea. I've only missed two of the classes. I'll start them again on Thursday.

Table 6–1. Tips for using behavioral activation

---

1. *Develop a collaborative relationship before trying behavioral activation.* Don't put the cart before the horse. Without good collaboration between patient and therapist, attempts to implement behavioral activation may fail. Part of the reason the patient may carry out the task is that he wants to work with you and can understand the reasons for making changes.
2. *Let the patient decide.* Although you can help guide the patient to actions that may be helpful, whenever possible ask him to make the choice.
3. *Judge the patient's readiness to change.* Before suggesting behavioral activation, gauge the patient's motivation and openness for taking this step. If the patient is not interested in doing things differently right now or is not ready to take action, defer the intervention. On the other hand, if the patient is open to start moving in a positive direction, capitalize on the moment.
4. *Prepare the patient for behavioral activation.* Lead up to the assignment with Socratic questions or other CBT interventions that pave the way for change. Try to ask questions that educate the patient about the benefits of taking action or that tap into motivations for doing things differently. One of the best questions is "How would this change make you feel?" If the answer is positive and the action stands a reasonable chance of being effective, the patient will be likely to follow through.
5. *Design assignments that are manageable.* Choose behavioral activation exercises that match the patient's energy level and capacity to change. Check out the details of the behavioral plan to be sure that it offers enough challenge but doesn't overload the patient. If needed, do brief coaching on ways to make the plan work out well.

The therapist had a solid therapeutic relationship with Georgine, knew her well, and was able to quickly implement a behavioral activation assignment that had potential for helping reverse her decline into deeper depression. The suggestions listed in Table 6–1 may help you implement effective behavioral activation plans.

Activity Scheduling

When fatigue and anhedonia progress to the point that patients feel exhausted and believe that they can experience little or no pleasure, they may benefit from activity scheduling. This systematic behavioral method is frequently used in CBT to reactivate people and help them find ways to improve their interest in life. Activity scheduling is most often used with patients who have moderate to severe depression. However, it can also have a place in the treatment of other patients who have difficulty organizing their days or engaging in productive activities. Activity scheduling focuses on activity assessment and increasing mastery and pleasure.

These methods, introduced in Juliana's case below, are described further following the case example.

Case Example

Juliana had severe depression and was a good candidate for activity scheduling. She was a 22-year-old, single Puerto Rican woman who had suffered the loss of her brother in a car accident a year before she started treatment with CBT. After her brother's death, Juliana dropped out of college to return home to comfort her parents. However, her own grief was intense and unrelenting. She was unable to make herself go back to school the following semester. Her parents understood Juliana's grief and did not force her to resume college or to get a job. Juliana's friends tried to be supportive for many months after her brother's death. But when she consistently rejected offers to go out to dinner and stopped returning phone calls, her friends eventually began to drift away.

Juliana was well cared for by her family. There was no real need for her to work, so no demands were placed on her. After about a year, her parents thought that Juliana had overcome much of the sadness from the loss of her brother. Yet there had been a distinct change in her behavior. She had developed a more serious demeanor, a preference for solitude, and a greater tendency toward introspection. Juliana's parents felt comfortable leaving her at home when they were at work or traveling out of town, because she appeared to be better. However, one evening her mother came home early from work and found Juliana preparing to hang herself in her closet.

After a brief hospitalization and initiation of pharmacotherapy, Juliana improved to the point that she could be referred to a cognitive-behavior therapist for outpatient treatment. Given the severity of her symptoms, one of the first treatment initiatives was to increase Juliana's activities so that she could benefit from the support of friends, feel better about her personal appearance, practice her social skills, and in general feel more like her old self. The intervention began with an assessment of her current level of activity, experiences that gave her pleasure, and the amount of mastery she felt over her world.

Activity Assessment

Because depressed patients tend to underreport positive experiences, emphasize negative perceptions, and focus more on failures than on successes, self-reports may not be as accurate as a log of activities kept for a week between therapy sessions. The weekly activity schedule form presented in Figure 6–1 can be assigned as homework but should be started in a session to ensure that the patient understands the concepts. The form is also available in a larger format at http://www.appi.org/pdf/wright. Beginning with the day of therapy, ask the patient to fill in her activities for each time block before the treatment session. Encourage her to write in the activities that actually occurred, no matter how mundane. For example, activities might include bathing, dressing, eating, traveling, talking with others on the phone or in person, watching television, and sleeping. If the patient has pronounced loss of energy or significant problems concentrating, it may be best to ask her to complete the schedule for only 1 day, or a part of a day. Inpatient applications of activity scheduling often employ a daily activity schedule instead of a weekly activity schedule (Wright et al. 1993).

To determine the impact of activities listed on a weekly or daily schedule, ask the patient to rate the degree of enjoyment experienced for each, as well as the sense of mastery or accomplishment that was associated with the activity. A scale of either 0–5 or 0–10 can be used (Beck et al. 1979, 1995; Wright et al. 2003). On a 0–10 scale, a rating of 0 on mastery suggests that the activity provided no experience of accomplishment, whereas a rating of 10 indicates a great sense of accomplishment. Some patients will give a low rating to simple tasks such as washing dishes or making themselves a cup of coffee because they do not consider those activities to be important. When this occurs, help the patient to understand the full range of the mastery and pleasure scales. Patients should try to give themselves credit for small accomplishments, because progress is generally made in small, incremental steps. Some simple tasks might receive high ratings for mastery. For example, after being immobilized by depression for some time, making breakfast can be a big feat and therefore might receive a rating of 8 or 9. Juliana's activity monitoring example is presented in Figure 6–2. For her, returning phone calls was an important accomplishment, since she had managed to avoid them for several months. Therefore, when she was able to make some calls, she gave herself a mastery rating of 8 on a 0–10 scale. In the past, Juliana would have rated returning phone calls only 4 for mastery because it took so little effort.

When symptoms of depression are moderate to severe, low ratings of pleasure should be expected for two reasons: 1) there is usually little involvement in activities that most people would consider highly pleasurable, and 2) the capacity for experiencing joy or pleasure is usually blunted. If an event that would normally make the patient laugh or smile elicits no more than an intellectual understanding that the stimulus was amusing, this event is likely to be given a low rating for pleasure. Help the patient reduce her expectations for feeling pleasure until the depression has improved. As an alternative to feeling disappointed with events and rating them 0, encourage the patient to at least give a rating of 1–3 if minimal pleasant feelings were experienced.

Weekly Activity Schedule

Instructions: Write down your activities for each hour and then rate them on a scale of 0–10 for mastery (**m**) or degree of accomplishment and for pleasure (**p**) or amount of enjoyment you experienced. A rating of 0 would mean that you had no sense of mastery or pleasure. A rating of 10 would mean that you experienced maximum mastery or pleasure.

	Sunday	Monday	Tuesday	Wednesday	Thursday	Friday	Saturday
8:00 A.M.							
9:00 A.M.							
10:00 A.M.							
11:00 A.M.							
12:00 P.M.							
1:00 P.M.							
2:00 P.M.							
3:00 P.M.							
4:00 P.M.							
5:00 P.M.							
6:00 P.M.							
7:00 P.M.							
8:00 P.M.							
9:00 P.M.							

Figure 6–1. Weekly activity schedule form.

Table 6–2. Activity monitoring

Are there distinct periods of time when the patient experiences pleasure?

What kinds of activities seem to give the patient pleasure?

Can these pleasurable activities be repeated on another day?

What activities appear to give the patient a sense of accomplishment?

Can these types of activities be scheduled for other days?

Are there certain times of day that appear to be low on mastery or pleasure?

What can be done to improve activity patterns during those times of day?

Do the ratings tend to be higher for activities that involve other people? If so, can social contact be increased?

What activities did the patient have in the past that have been stopped or reduced? Are there opportunities for rekindling interest in these activities?

Are there any types of activities (e.g., exercise, music, spiritual involvement, art, crafts, reading, volunteer work, cooking) that the patient is ignoring but that may interest her? Is she open to considering adding new or different activities to her weekly schedule?

Juliana gave having dinner with her parents a rating of only 1 for pleasure. When questioned about what elements of dinner she had enjoyed, she listed the comfort of being with her mother, the mashed potatoes with butter, and the banana pudding—a childhood favorite—she had had for dessert. When queried about why three different enjoyable things resulted in a rating of only 1 for pleasure, she reconsidered the rating and raised it to a 4. It was hard for her not to be conscious of her brother's absence during family meals, and thinking about his loss usually lowered her mood. But when she gave more consideration to the positive parts of the meal, it seemed more enjoyable overall. With this in mind, Juliana rerated some of the other activities on her schedule and raised their pleasure ratings accordingly.

The questions in Table 6–2 are designed to help you evaluate and change patients' activity levels.

Juliana's activity monitoring exercise revealed a pattern of greatest pleasure when she was involved in activities outside the house or when she made an attempt to connect with friends (making phone calls). She gave one of her highest ratings for pleasure to walking her dog. In contrast, the lowest pleasure ratings were given to being home alone with nothing to do. Because her involvement in productive activities had fallen to such a low level, her ratings of mastery were usually minimal. Mastery ratings also appeared to be influenced by her lack of goals for the future. Juliana complained that her life had no meaning. She had limited household responsibilities, was no longer in school, did not have a job, had lost touch with her friends, and had no clear prospects for becoming more involved in life. Thus she needed to find activities or commitments that would give her a sense of purpose and fulfillment.

Weekly Activity Schedule

Instructions: Write down your activities for each hour and then rate them on a scale of 0–10 for mastery (m) or degree of accomplishment and for pleasure (p) or amount of enjoyment you experienced. A rating of 0 would mean that you had no sense of mastery or pleasure. A rating of 10 would mean that you experienced maximum mastery or pleasure.

	Sunday	Monday	Tuesday	Wednesday	Thursday	Friday	Saturday
8:00 A.M.	Wake up m-2 Get dressed p-0				Wake up m-3 Get dressed p-1		Wake up m-2 Get dressed p-1
9:00 A.M.	Church with parents m-3 p-4				Walk the dog m-5 p-7		Walk the dog m-4 Breakfast p-5
10:00 A.M.		Wake up m-3 Get dressed p-1	Wake up m-3 Get dressed p-1	Wake up m-3 Get dressed p-1	Therapy m-7 p-6		
11:00 A.M.		Walk the dog m-4 Breakfast p-6	Walk the dog m-4 p-5	Walk the dog m-4 p-5		Wake up m-3 Get dressed p-1	
12:00 P.M.	Lunch with parents m-4 p-2					Walk the dog m-5 p-6	Clean my room m-6 p-3
1:00 P.M.			Lunch m-2 p-2	Lunch m-2 p-2			
2:00 P.M.	Read newspaper m-4 p-2	Bring in the mail m-3 p-1	Bring in the mail m-3 p-1	Bring in the mail m-3 p-1	Bring in the mail m-4 p-2	Bring in the mail m-4 p-3	Hand wash laundry m-7 p-4

Figure 6–2. Juliana's activity schedule.

	Sunday	Monday	Tuesday	Wednesday	Thursday	Friday	Saturday
3:00 P.M.	Read magazine m-4 p-4						
4:00 P.M.		Watch Oprah m-1 p-3	Watch Oprah m-1 p-3	Watch Oprah m-1 p-3	Watch Oprah m-1 p-3	Buy food for dinner m-6 p-2	
5:00 P.M.						Walk the dog m-5 p-7	Walk the dog m-5 p-7
6:00 P.M.	Walk the dog m-4 p-5	Dinner with parents m-2 p-4	Dinner with parents m-3 p-4	Dinner with parents m-3 p-4	Dinner with parents m-3 p-4	Dinner alone m-5 p-3	Cook/eat dinner alone m-5 p-4
7:00 P.M.	Dinner with parents m-2 p-4	Walk the dog m-4 p-6	Walk the dog m-4 p-6	Walk the dog m-4 p-5	Walk the dog m-5 p-7		
8:00 P.M.	TV w/Mom m-2 p-4	Make phone calls m-8 p-5		TV w/Mom m-2 p-5		TV alone m-2 p-2	TV alone m-2 p-3
9:00 P.M.							

Figure 6–2. Juliana's activity schedule.

Another strategy for use of the activity scheduling technique is to ask the patient to rate his mood on a 0–10 scale while engaging in each activity. In Video Illustration 12, Dr. Thase examines Ed's mood ratings for each activity to help explain how events can affect mood. Activities were planned that had the highest potential for improving mood. In Ed's case, one of these was to resume singing in the shower. Although to someone who is not experiencing anhedonia such ordinary activities may seem routine or of limited consequence, they can provide keys for helping depressed persons break out of negative behavioral patterns and begin to climb out of depression.

▶ **Video Illustration 12.** Activity Scheduling: Dr. Thase and Ed

Increasing Mastery and Pleasure

If you have determined that there are deficits in experiences of mastery or pleasure in the course of a patient's day-to-day life, you can help make improvements by scheduling activities between sessions that will make him feel good about himself. Begin by generating a list of pleasurable activities. Include the ones from the monitoring exercise that had the highest ratings of pleasure. Also brainstorm with the patient to list some new ideas that may be worth trying (see the questions in Table 6–2). Then collaboratively determine which activities to add to the person's daily routine. Select specific times and write them on the schedule as a plan for the following week.

Next, use the activity monitoring exercise to help you determine the types of activities that seem to produce feelings of mastery. For example, Juliana's activity schedule (see Figure 6–2) shows higher mastery scores when she was responsible for making her own dinner and when she did her own chores. You can recommend that the patient continue existing activities that are high on mastery or modify current activities to increase their value to the patient. If the patient has completed a goal list, efforts toward completion of any of the stated goals can be added to the activity schedule.

After completing the schedule, elicit the patient's predictions for success in changing his level of activity. Evaluate any negative automatic thoughts that are reported. Before going on to another agenda item, ask about any factors that could interfere with the patient's ability to follow the activity schedule as planned. Devise a strategy for overcoming any projected obstacles to adherence and also create a backup plan in case unforeseen factors keep the patient from engaging in any of the planned activities. Armed with this information, assign the new schedule for the following week and ask the patient to rate each event for mastery and pleasure. Review the plan at the next session and modify it as needed. Usually activity scheduling is used in the early parts of therapy and can be discontinued when the patient is able to initiate pleasurable and achievement-oriented activities spontaneously. However, we sometimes use activity scheduling later in therapy when there are persistent problems with anhedonia, organizing effective behavioral plans, or procrastination.

Learning Exercise 6–1. Activity Scheduling

1. Complete at least 1 day of an activity schedule for your own life. Review the ratings of mastery and pleasure.

2. Practice introducing an activity schedule in a role-play exercise with a colleague.

3. Use activity scheduling in your clinical practice.

Graded Task Assignments

Graded task assignment (GTA) is a method for making overwhelming tasks seem more manageable by breaking them down into smaller and more easily accomplished pieces. GTA can be used in conjunction with activity scheduling to increase mastery experiences and is particularly helpful when patients have fallen behind on chores (e.g., household maintenance or yard work), when they have put off difficult tasks that have looming deadlines (e.g., paying bills or filing taxes), or when goals they wish to accomplish are complicated and require lengthy efforts (e.g., getting in shape, earning a General Educational Development [GED] certificate or college degree, filing for divorce). If the perceived magnitude of tasks has kept patients from taking action, GTA may be the answer.

Begin GTA by eliciting patients' perceptions of the tasks that require attention. Listen for negative automatic thoughts and evaluate their validity before beginning GTA. Catastrophic thoughts and black-and-white thinking can interfere with initiative. Ask patients to write down their modified thoughts and to review this cognitive analysis before initiating behavioral exercises. Suggest that they hold on to this written record as a handy reminder in case negative thoughts return. Below, an example from the treatment of Robert illustrates the value of eliciting automatic thoughts about taking behavioral actions.

Case Example

Therapist: When you think about filing your taxes, what goes through your mind?

Robert: I go blank. I don't know where to start.

Therapist: Take a moment and imagine yourself at home and seeing a commercial for a tax service on television. What would you be thinking?

Robert: I feel this tightness in my throat. I want to change the channel.

Therapist: Change the channel because you imagine what?

Robert: I know I have to file my taxes. I didn't turn them in last year, and I know the IRS [Internal Revenue Service] is going to go after me if I turn in this year's report. I don't know how to get started. I don't have the forms. I can't ask anyone else to help because I would have to tell them that I never filed taxes last year. That would be too embarrassing. It's all too much for me right now.

Therapist: So when you are reminded that you have to file your taxes, you get pretty upset.

Robert: You got that right.

Therapist: And when you get upset, what happens to your motivation to begin working on the taxes?

Robert: I don't want to deal with it. I put it off for another day.

Therapist: If you thought you had the ability to handle the stress of doing the taxes, would you want to start tackling the problem?

Robert: I have to do something about it.

Therapist: What would happen if we could find a way to make it easier for you?

Robert: If it were easier, I think I might be able to handle it. But it's not easy.

Therapist: I think I know a way to help.

Robert was overwhelmed by the thought of filing taxes, partly because he was uncertain where to begin. He had also made a number of assumptions about the reactions others would have if he asked for help. The therapist started working with Robert by modifying the belief that he couldn't ask for help. When this was accomplished, they were able to break the task down into smaller parts and make a schedule for their completion.

The behavioral component of GTA involves listing the parts of a task and then placing them in a logical order. Because there are usually many ways to tackle an uncompleted task, it often helps to discuss several possible approaches before creating a specific action plan.

Robert thought it might be best to begin by finding someone to help him with his taxes. His sister, Celeste, thought it would be better for Robert to organize his materials and collect the proper tax forms before asking someone for help. His mother, Brenda, suggested he start by calling the IRS to find out if it would be better to turn in last year's tax return first or work on the one for this year. After discussing these options with his therapist, Robert decided to follow his first inclination and ask for assistance. He was so overwhelmed with the task, he did not think he could initiate things on his own. So he decided to ask Celeste for help as his first step.

The remaining steps involved finding the materials he had at home, organizing them, downloading the appropriate form from the IRS Web site, scheduling time with Celeste to begin filling out the forms, completing the forms, and calling the IRS to discuss last year's taxes. Because he wasn't certain about the order of the steps and thought it was possible that there were other things he needed to do, Robert asked Celeste for advice about the order of the remaining tasks and for suggestions about any other steps that might be needed.

When patients report on their progress at subsequent therapy sessions, you should praise their efforts and inquire about how their actions made them feel about themselves. Reinforce the cognitive-behavioral model, explaining once again that positive changes in action will help to improve mood, strengthen self-esteem, and create optimism about future efforts. Ask about their motivation to take on the next step and elicit and modify negative thoughts if necessary. After the first few items from the GTA have been assigned, some patients may feel enough momentum building to follow through with the other tasks without assistance from the therapist. Others will require continued coaching from the therapist to maintain progress. As energy and motivation levels return to normal, GTA may no longer be needed to initiate activity.

There will be times when GTA is not successful. A common reason is that the steps are too complicated for the patient to accomplish or require more energy than the patient possesses. In these cases, complex tasks must be broken down into small substeps. You will need to match the task to the energy level and the time available to the patient. Another common reason that GTA fails is that the person is flooded with negative automatic thoughts that discourage or interfere with his taking action. When tasks are difficult, initial attempts to carry them out may be less than completely successful. The person who is prone to black-and-white thinking may not give herself credit for progress made toward a goal. Instead, partial success is viewed as failure. When designing a GTA intervention, caution should be taken to keep each step within the capacity of the patient. When in doubt, it is better to make a task too easy to accomplish than too difficult.

In Video Illustration 13, Dr. Thase uses a combination of GTA and activity scheduling to help Ed make plans for completing a critical work assignment. Ed is a newspaper writer who is facing a deadline for a project. He has been slowed by depression, but he still has many strengths that can be organized in a graded task plan. Breaking down each activity into more discrete behaviors and planning the time for their execution increased the chances that Ed would be able to bring this project to a successful conclusion.

▶ **Video Illustration 13.** Graded Task Assignment: Dr. Thase and Ed

Behavioral Rehearsal

Any behavioral plan that you want the patient to complete outside therapy can first be rehearsed in a treatment session to 1) check on the patient's ability to carry out the activity, 2) practice behavioral skills, 3) give feedback to the patient, 4) spot potential roadblocks, and 5) coach the patient on ways to ensure that the plan will have a positive outcome. The next case illustration shows how behavioral rehearsal might be used to help a patient be assertive in an interpersonal situation.

> Bernice was a single mother with a 5-year-old boy, Ben, who could be difficult to manage at times. Bernice and her parents felt bad for Ben because his father had left them when Ben was just a toddler. So they doted on the child to try to compensate for his father's absence. Ben was quite smart and had figured out that if his mother would not give him what he wanted, his grandfather would. For example, Bernice told him, "No, you can't jump on the bed," but Ben begged, "Please, please, please," and began to cry. Bernice tried to stand firm, but she noticed later that her father would allow Ben to jump on his bed even though he knew that Bernice did not allow such behavior. In the past Bernice would eventually give in to Ben's pleadings, but she had made efforts to set more consistent limits. She needed her father to do the same, but she did not know how to talk with him about it without hurting his feelings or putting him on the defensive. So she said nothing and allowed her son to continue to manipulate the situation and learn a double standard for behavior.

Confronting someone about his or her actions is not easy to do, especially when that person may not take it well and when the consequences for hurting that person's feelings seem great. Bernice was in that type of situation with her father. She wanted to assert herself in disciplining Ben but was concerned about putting a strain on her relationship with her father. After sorting through the pros and cons of speaking up on an important point, it can be helpful for patients to practice what they are going to say and receive feedback from the therapist. This is one of the commonly used applications of behavioral rehearsal. These steps can help people formulate and rehearse delivery of a difficult message.

An Example of Behavioral Rehearsal: Being Assertive in Communicating With Others

1. *Start with a general idea.* Ask the patient to describe what she would ideally like to communicate to another person if the circumstances allowed.
2. *Help the patient shape her idea into a clear statement.* Discourage beating around the bush or any language that is vague or ambiguous. Ask the patient to articulate the message, and then give feedback to the patient on what you heard in the statement. Then modify the message until it communicates specifically what the patient wants to say and has a reasonable likelihood of achieving the desired results:

   > Bernice began with the statement, "Dad, I want to talk about Ben's habit of begging for things. You know how he can be. I don't think we should always give him what he wants." Although this statement describes part of the problem, it avoids telling her father directly that he is the one who needs to change his behavior. When she tried this approach in the past, her father responded with "OK, honey. I agree." After working further on her communication skills, Bernice came up with a message that conveyed her main points: "Dad, I want to talk with you about my new strategy for handling Ben when he tries to get away with things we don't like him to do—for example, jumping on the bed. I want to say 'No' and to stick with it even if he whines or begs. He needs to learn to respond to my words at this young age so that when he gets older, we have already set a precedent for following my instructions. But I need your help to make it work. Whenever you hear me set limits with Ben, I need you to back me up and treat him in the same way, even when you disagree with me or think I am being too hard on him. Are you willing to do that?"

3. *Use the "good news, bad news, good news" method of communication.* Encourage the patient to begin the conversation with a positive statement or compliment to the listener. She should follow this with the assertive or confrontational component of the message and follow it up with another positive statement. Examples of positive introductory statements are "Thank you for agreeing to meet with me; I appreciate your time" and "You are doing a good job with _____; I want you to know that I appreciate all you do for me." Examples of positive closing statements are "Thank you for listening to me; I appreciate your willingness to hear me out" and "I knew I could count on you to listen; I feel so much better after talking with you."

4. *Role-play the interaction with the patient.* After a statement has been formulated, prepare for a behavioral rehearsal by asking the patient to describe how the listener is likely to respond. Elicit a best-case scenario, a worst-case scenario, and the most likely scenario. Role-play the best-case scenario to give the patient a chance to practice. Provide feedback on the delivery. Practice the worst-case scenario. Challenge the patient to stick by her statement despite your negative reaction as you role-play the listener. Help the patient prepare and practice her response. Then role-play the most likely scenario.

5. *Elicit the patient's predictions for the event.* For any negative prediction, brainstorm ways to prevent the interaction from going badly. Ideas might include careful selection of the time and place for the interaction. Make a plan for recovering from an interaction that goes badly:

> Bernice knew it was never a good idea to bring up difficult topics with her father when he was hungry or when he was in a hurry. She planned to talk with him after lunch on Saturday, when he would be most relaxed and when Ben would be taking a nap. If it went badly, she would apologize for upsetting him, thank him for being such a good grandfather, and suggest they talk about it again later.

Behavioral rehearsal has many applications in CBT. For example, you might practice breathing training for reducing anxiety, exposure protocols for overcoming panic and avoidance, or strategies for stopping compulsive rituals (see Chapter 7, "Behavioral Methods II: Reducing Anxiety and Breaking Patterns of Avoidance"). Behaviors that may enhance adherence to medication regimens (e.g., using effective communication with the prescribing physician, organizing a complex medication regimen, implementing a reminder system) could also be rehearsed in a treatment session. Other opportunities for using behavioral rehearsal might include role-playing a plan worked out in a problem-solving exercise (see Learning Exercise 6–2 below) or practicing skills for managing social anxiety (e.g., how to make small talk).

Learning Exercise 6–2.   Task Completion

1. In a role-playing exercise with a colleague, target a challenging or difficult task.

2. First practice using the graded task assignment method to work out a plan to complete the task.

3. Then use behavioral rehearsal to build skills or spot potential problems in carrying out the plan.

4. Role-play another behavioral rehearsal exercise.

Problem Solving

When people have difficulties solving their problems, it may be partly due to either a *performance* deficit or a *skill* deficit. Those with performance deficits possess adequate problem-solving skills but—due to depression, anxiety, extreme stress, or feelings of helplessness—have difficulty accessing and utilizing those skills. In contrast, people with skill deficits may be unable to analyze the nature of a problem and cannot seem to come up with reasonable ideas to solve it. Individuals with skill deficits often have had trouble solving problems in many different areas of their lives or have repeatedly chosen solutions that have failed or have made matters worse. People with performance deficits can be helped by identifying and modifying, whenever possible, the factors that keep them from using their existing skills. However, patients with skill deficits may require basic training in problem-resolution methods.

Working With Problem-Solving Performance Deficits

Some of the more common factors that interfere with effective problem solving are listed in Table 6–3. This list includes obstacles that may be associated with the symptoms of a mental or physical illness. For example, depression often impairs concentration and interferes with the cognitive functioning needed to solve problems. Other roadblocks occur when patients do not have the resources to properly address their problems (e.g., financial, intellectual, or physical limitations) or when they search for ideal or perfect solutions when such standards are not attainable.

Cognitive Impairment

When reduced attention span and impaired concentration keep a person from being able to focus on a problem, stimulus control measures may be needed. Stimulus control procedures involve arranging the physical environment so that stimuli that might interfere with accomplishing a goal are limited or avoided, while environmental factors that can facilitate goal attainment are identified and promoted. If concentration is a prob-

Table 6–3.   Obstacles to effective problem solving

Cognitive impairment	Poor concentration, slowed thinking, impaired decision making
Emotional overload	Feeling overwhelmed, dysphoric, anxious
Cognitive distortions	Negative automatic thoughts, cognitive errors (e.g., catastrophizing, all-or-nothing thinking, magnification), hopelessness, self-criticism
Avoidance	Procrastination, forgetfulness
Social factors	Contradictory advice from others, criticism, lack of support
Practical problems	Insufficient time, limited resources, problem being beyond control
Strategy factors	Trying to find the perfect solution, looking for one overall solution that will solve several related problems

lem, environmental noise and confusion can distract the person from a task, whereas peace and quiet can facilitate completion of the task.

Case Example

Jonathan was so concerned that he would not be able to pay all his bills that he was losing sleep, was distracted at work by worries about his finances, and was experiencing frequent headaches. He needed to solve the problem by figuring out what bills needed to be paid, which ones could be delayed, when they were due, and the total amount that he owed. He had been working on his bills while sitting at the kitchen table after dinner, but he had not been able to concentrate well enough to get the job done. When his therapist asked what was happening around him while he tried to pay bills, Jonathan described a noisy dining room table with the dinner dishes being cleared by his wife. The television was on, and his children were watching a comedy and laughing hysterically. Although he wished they would be quiet, he knew they were just kids, and the sound of their laughter did him some good. His oldest daughter was usually on the phone in the kitchen. He never listened in on her conversations, but he did worry that she might be talking to an older boy who gave her a ride home from time to time. The therapist concluded that Jonathan's environment was not conducive to concentration and problem solving.

Stimulus control can facilitate concentration and problem solving by reducing distractions and by creating an environment that makes it more likely that the goal will be achieved.

Jonathan needed a place to work that was free of extraneous visual and auditory stimuli. He needed a physical space with enough room to sort through his bills; the tools to accomplish the task such as paper, pencils, and a calculator; and enough time and energy to complete the task. These conditions were hard to come by during the workweek because his house was small, there were no quiet places to work on the bills, and he was always tired at the end of the day. When he was not depressed, Jonathan could tune everyone out and get the job done. But now his concentration was poor, and he didn't realize that his environment was part of the problem. After the therapist explained the principles of stimulus control, Jonathan concluded that he needed to set aside time early on Saturday morning to pay his bills. He chose a time before the children would be awake and before his wife would start to make breakfast.

Stimuli that interfere with concentration can be visual as well as auditory. Creating a quiet time with few auditory distractions can improve concentration, as can creating an environment with few visual distractions. These efforts are particularly helpful for people who work at a desk piled with materials. To control visual stimuli, have the patient clear the space, organize piles of materials, and work on one thing at a time.

Emotional Overload

Efforts to diminish the intensity of emotion can also facilitate problem solving. Cognitive restructuring methods described below under "Cognitive Distortions" are among the primary problem-solving techniques used to reduce distracting or painful emotions. A variety of other ideas can be tried such as relaxation exercises, prayer, listening to music, physical exercise, massage, yoga, or self-care behaviors that induce a temporary feeling of well-being. These might include going for a walk, taking a warm bath, eating a favorite food, or sitting in a garden. The goal is to reduce tension—not to encourage avoidance of the task. When the person feels calmer, he can begin to tackle the problem. If he becomes overwhelmed again, a brief break should be taken to reduce tension.

Cognitive Distortions

The key to using cognitive restructuring methods (see Chapter 5, "Working With Automatic Thoughts") for problem solving is teaching patients how to carry the lessons of therapy into real-life situations. After learning in treatment sessions how to recognize negative automatic thoughts and how to correct cognitive distortions, patients can start to apply this knowledge toward conceptualizing and coping with their environmental problems. A good illustration of the usefulness of cognitive restructuring is the application of methods for spotting and correcting cognitive errors. Patients with depression may magnify the seriousness of their problems, minimize their resources or strengths for coping with the difficulty, take excessive blame for the situation (i.e., personalization), and give global meaning to a problem when it can have circumscribed significance. If the person can recognize and revise these cognitive errors, she will be able to develop a clearer picture of the challenges she faces and the opportunities she has to solve the problem.

Avoidance

Techniques described elsewhere in this chapter (see "Activity Scheduling" and "Graded Task Assignments" above) can be used effectively to help people overcome avoidance. In Chapter 7, "Behavioral Methods II: Reducing Anxiety and Breaking Patterns of Avoidance," we discuss other behavioral methods that can help patients cope with avoidance problems associated with anxiety disorders. All of these behavioral methods involve organizing a plan that is systematic, that overcomes helplessness or paralyzing fear, and that utilizes gradual or stepwise methods of taking action.

Social Factors

When people seek out advice from significant others, they may receive a variety of suggestions that have the potential of being helpful. However, advice can also be conflicting, ineffective, or harmful. To help the patient sort out the advice received, you can recommend that he analyze the pros and cons of each suggestion made by others, as well as any ideas that he has come up with himself. Craft a solution that offers the most advantages and the fewest disadvantages. If the patient is uncertain whether a significant other will be offended by the patient's not accepting advice, encourage the patient to check out this possibility with that person. Some people who are asked for advice will feel a personal investment in solving the problem and may therefore be more forceful with their suggestions. The potential for disappointing others by not taking their advice can create a new problem for the indecisive patient with low self-esteem. Therefore, you may need to coach the patient in skills for communicating effectively with these people.

    Some of the most difficult barriers to problem solving are 1) lack of social support; 2) criticism and disparagement from family members, friends, or others; and 3) active efforts of other people to block problem resolution. Examples of the latter would be a spouse in a divorce case who refuses mediation and appears determined to cause the most distress possible to the patient; a child who continues to use illicit drugs despite intense efforts by the patient to help him get treatment; and a boss who is extremely critical and is unwilling to give the patient any constructive ideas for meeting his expectations. Some of these types of problems cannot be solved easily, if at all. Therefore, the strategy should include a realistic assessment of the chances of any change occurring, the resources the patient may have to respond to the challenge, and alternative ideas that may not have been tried previously. Advice from an expert may be needed. The patient may also benefit from reading books, viewing videos, attending support groups, consulting a counselor in an employee assistance program, or using other methods to get ideas on how to manage the situation.

Practical Problems

When functioning has declined during a lengthy episode of depression, it is not unusual to find that the patient has developed significant practical problems, especially when symptoms have been severe enough to interfere with his ability to sustain employment. Financial difficulties can quickly mount. Medical problems can be neglected due to lack of health insurance. Housing may be in jeopardy because of an inability to continue making rent or mortgage payments. The desperation communicated by patients in these situations can be disheartening for therapists. If your cognitions begin to echo the patient's hopelessness, you can lose your ability to be objective and creative with problem solving. Therefore, when faced with a patient with limited resources to solve his problems, it is important to process your own negative automatic thoughts about the bleakness of the situation.

If you can retain a reasonable degree of optimism that solutions can be found, you will be more likely to help the patient persevere. Help him brainstorm ideas for facing the problem. If ideas do not come easily, ask the patient what he would have done about this same problem at a time in his life when he was not depressed. Or ask him what a thoughtful and supportive advisor might recommend. Don't allow the patient to discount solutions as quickly as they are generated. Keep a running list of ideas, and wait until the brainstorming has been completed to evaluate their potential.

When people are depressed, they often feel alone in their misery. They forget that there are people in their world who could provide assistance if they knew there was a need. Most patients would agree to help others in similar situations. If solutions considered by the patient do not include asking for help from family, friends, faith communities, or social service agencies, encourage him to think about these possibilities. Embarrassment or pride can keep people from asking for help. But when times are desperate, the patient may need to temporarily forgo a self-reliant style of problem solving.

Strategy Factors

When depressed or anxious, some people discard obvious solutions because they seem too simple. Or they look for solutions that are perfectly thought out or are guaranteed to succeed. Sometimes they look for the magic solution that will resolve several issues simultaneously.

Case Example

Olivia lost her job and had been looking for a replacement. She had two children in elementary school. The three of them lived with her elderly grandmother, who had recently developed some health problems. Olivia needed to make enough money to support her children, but she also needed a job that was close to their school so that she could get to them in the event of an emergency. She needed a compassionate boss who would allow her extra time at lunch to look in on her grandmother. Olivia did not want to hire a home health aide to assist her grandmother, and she preferred to put her children in an after-school program rather than in private day care. A job near the school would make it possible for her to meet her children at the time the program closed. The children's father finished work earlier in the day, but Olivia did not trust him to pick them up on time. Olivia had marketable skills and could find a job in the larger city a little farther from her home. She could ask her sister to help with the grandmother rather than take on the full responsibility for her care, but she felt obligated to do it herself because her grandmother had been so helpful to her in times of need. Thinking about how to make all the pieces come together exhausted Olivia. As a result, she gave up reading the want ads and immersed herself in doing household chores.

The answer to a dilemma like Olivia's is to help her change problem-solving strategies. Instead of trying to find one large solution, work with her to sort out the problems and find a solution that covers as many areas as possible. Draw out her underlying problem-solving skills, identify key resources and supports, and coach her on ways of simplifying the plan or taking it one step at a time.

Working With Deficits in Problem-Solving Skills

Problem-solving skills are usually learned during childhood and refined during early adulthood when one is grappling with life transitions and psychosocial stressors. If good role models were available, the person has probably learned by watching these people systematically work through problems and generate solutions. Furthermore, if the patient had early life experiences in which she was able to solve problems effectively, she may have developed the self-confidence and competence needed to take on future difficulties. Unfortunately, patients may not have acquired effective problem-solving skills—perhaps because they had ineffective role models, they were protected by parents who solved problems for them, or they were too depressed when they were growing up to build these skills. When the patient has had limited experience in effectively conceptualizing and managing problems, CBT can be used to teach basic skills for problem resolution.

One useful way of helping patients gain these skills is to model problem-solving strategies in treatment sessions. For example, the steps listed in Table 6–4 might be used to assist patients with organizing a plan to tackle one of the difficulties on their problem list. The suggested structure helps patients organize their thoughts, approach the problem in an objective fashion, and see the process through to completion.

Table 6–4. Problem-solving steps

1. Slow down and sort it out.
2. Pick a target.
3. Define the problem accurately.
4. Generate solutions.
5. Select the most reasonable solution.
6. Implement the plan.
7. Evaluate the outcome and repeat the steps if needed.

---

1. *Slow down and sort it out.* When patients describe their psychosocial difficulties in treatment sessions, they may jump from topic to topic. As they describe one problem, another comes to mind. Without realizing it, they present a disjointed list of issues, all of which may seem equally pressing and stressful. They may see links between the problems and layers of complexity that combine the facts of the situation, the people involved, the deeper meanings behind them, and implications for the future. When problems are reported in this fashion, the notion of resolving these difficulties can seem distant or hopeless.

    The first order of business is to slow down the process by defining the number and magnitude of problems and the urgency of resolving them. You can ask the patient to keep a written list of problems in his treatment notebook. After the patient is finished recording the problems, ask him to summarize by reading back the list. Empathize with him about how distressing it must be to face so many challenges at one time. Then go on with the next steps in the problem-solving process.

2. *Pick a target.* Teach the patient how to organize the list by prioritizing problems. For example, ask him to cross off the list any problem that has already been resolved or is currently dormant. Next ask the patient to eliminate items over which he has no control or problems that belong to others and cannot be resolved by him. Help the patient to separate the remaining items into difficulties that must be addressed in the near future and ones whose resolution could be delayed for some time. Then ask the patient to consider the most pressing problems and place them in order of priority based on importance or urgency. The final part of this step is to select one item from the top two or three as the beginning target for therapy.

3. *Define the problem accurately.* If problems can be stated in clear terms, patients may be more likely to generate specific solutions. You can assist patients with defining problems accurately by teaching them the principles of goal and agenda setting described in Chapter 4, "Structuring and Educating." It may also be helpful to ask questions that help patients sharpen their definitions. Examples of these types of questions would be "How could you define this problem so that you would know if you were making progress to cope with it?" "How could you state this problem in just a few words so that other people would know exactly what you are facing?" and "There seem to be lots of different issues involved in this problem....How could you define the problem so that you can zero in on the central issue?"

4. *Generate solutions.* There are usually many different ways to solve any given problem. People sometimes lock onto the first solution that comes to mind and become convinced that it is the only way to cope. However, their selected solution may not be practical, effective, or possible to implement. Finding it difficult to change directions, they may flounder or completely give up on attempting to resolve the problem. Try to help the patient learn to be creative in looking for solutions. For example, use the brainstorming technique or ask Socratic questions that stimulate creativity. Patients might consider ideas such as a) utilizing the assistance of others; b) doing research by reading, checking the Internet, or searching for community resources; c) delaying implementation of the plan; and d) considering not solving the problem at all but learning to live with it. It also may help to add your own suggestions to the list, but only after the patient has come up with a number of possibilities.

5. *Select the most reasonable solution.* Help the patient eliminate from the list any solutions that the patient concludes are unrealistic, are not likely to be useful, cannot be easily implemented at present, or could cause more problems than they solve. Ask the patient to pick the so-

lution that she thinks is most likely to succeed and that she is willing to implement. Sometimes patients will make a choice that in your best judgment will fail. Instead of discouraging the patient by telling her your opinion, help her choose one or two other possibilities and then evaluate the advantages and disadvantages of each. As the solutions are compared, the most appropriate choice usually becomes evident. Retain the original list of options in case they are needed at a later date.

6. *Implement the plan.* Once a solution has been selected, increase the chances of success by having the patient select a day and time to try out her plan. Role play or rehearsal methods can be used to coach patients on problem-solving skills. Troubleshoot by inquiring about circumstances that could interfere with success, and develop a plan for coping if these problems should occur.

7. *Evaluate the outcome and repeat the steps if needed.* Despite great planning, solutions will sometimes fail. There may be unforeseen circumstances or elements of the problem that were not fully considered. When there are difficulties in carrying out a plan, help patients evaluate their automatic thoughts about their efforts to solve the problem, and assist them with correcting any distortions. In addition, review the manner in which the solution was implemented, to determine whether further skills training may be required. Revise the plan if necessary, and try again.

Summary

When patients have problems with reduced activity levels, low energy, lack of interest, and poor task completion, behavioral methods can help restore healthy functioning. The easiest technique to implement is behavioral activation—a simple exercise in which the therapist and patient choose one or two concrete actions that appear to be immediately doable and are likely to improve mood or self-esteem. Activity scheduling, a more systematic method of recording and shaping behavior, is often quite useful when patients are experiencing moderate to severe reductions in energy and interest. Another behavioral technique, graded task assignment, can help patients organize a step-by-step plan to manage difficult or challenging tasks or to reverse patterns of procrastination and avoidance.

Behavioral rehearsal is commonly used in CBT to help patients develop action plans, build skills, and spot potential roadblocks in advance. This technique involves practicing behavioral methods in treatment sessions and then carrying out the plan for homework. Problem solving is another key behavioral method for helping patients cope with their stressors. Although some patients have good basic problem-solving skills and need help only in overcoming obstacles to using these strengths, others may need to be educated on the principles of effective problem solving. The behavioral methods described in this chapter can have a positive impact on a patient's activity level, mood, effectiveness in managing challenges, and hope for the future.

References

Beck AT, Rush AJ, Shaw BF, et al: Cognitive Therapy of Depression. New York, Guilford, 1979

Beck AT, Greenberg RL, Beck J: Coping With Depression. Bala Cynwyd, PA, Beck Institute for Cognitive Therapy and Research, 1995

Wright JH, Thase ME, Beck AT, et al (eds): Cognitive Therapy With Inpatients: Developing a Cognitive Milieu. New York, Guilford, 1993

Wright JH, Beck AT, Thase M: Cognitive therapy, in The American Psychiatric Publishing Textbook of Clinical Psychiatry, 4th Edition. Edited by Hales RE, Yudofsky SC. Washington, DC, American Psychiatric Publishing, 2003, pp 1245–1284

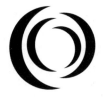

7

Behavioral Methods II

Reducing Anxiety and Breaking Patterns of Avoidance

The cognitive and behavioral features of anxiety disorders—unrealistic fears of objects or situations, overestimates of risk or danger, underestimates of ability to manage or cope with feared stimuli, and repeated patterns of avoidance—are outlined in Chapter 1, "Basic Principles of Cognitive-Behavior Therapy." We turn now to explaining the theoretical background for using behavioral techniques in anxiety disorders and to discussing specific methods for overcoming problems such as phobia, panic, and posttraumatic stress disorder (PTSD). The focus is on general principles and techniques that can be used for many different types of anxiety disorders.

Behavioral Analysis of Anxiety Disorders

The behavioral methods typically used in cognitive-behavior therapy (CBT) for anxiety disorders were originally derived from the learning theory model that shaped the early development of behavior therapy (see Chapter 1, "Basic Principles of Cognitive-Behavior Therapy"). As behavior therapy and cognitive therapy matured, these two approaches were merged into the comprehensive cognitive-behavioral approach that we describe in this book. To explain the rationale for behavioral methods for anxiety, we briefly detail the learning theory concepts that underlie contemporary use of these interventions.

Patients with anxiety disorders usually report intense subjective experiences of fear accompanied by physical symptoms of arousal when exposed to a threatening stimulus. For example, if a person who has a phobia for heights is facing the prospect of climbing a tall ladder, he may have anxiety-provoking automatic thoughts (e.g., "I'll pass out…I'll fall…I can't stand it…I have to get down right away") and intense emotions and physiological activation (e.g., anxiety, sweating, fast heartbeat, quickened breathing, clamminess). In learning theory, the feared object or circumstance is the *stimulus* (S), and the reaction of anxiety elicited by the stimulus is the *response* (R), as follows:

$$S \longrightarrow R$$

The original stimulus that frightened the person is called the *unconditioned stimulus* (UCS). Examples of unconditioned stimuli include places where a person first had a panic attack; events that were traumatic, such as an assault or a serious accident; or people who caused the individual hurt or distress. The original fearful response to the UCS is called the *unconditioned response* (UCR). Things that remind the patient of these stimuli can also elicit a fear response. The term *stimulus generalization* is used to describe the triggering of anxiety by these associated reminders. In the language of learning theory, these reminders are called *conditioned stimuli*, and the anxiety that they elicit is called the *conditioned response* (CR). Each time the conditioned stimulus (CS) is presented, the CR occurs, as follows:

$$CS \longrightarrow CR$$

In persons with anxiety disorders, the emotional and physiological responses to feared stimuli are usually so aversive that the sufferer will do whatever is necessary to avoid experiencing these situations again. Thus, persons with social phobia will stay away from events or places where they may feel exposed to social pressures; those with simple phobias will avoid heights, closed spaces, elevators, or other triggers for their anxiety; patients with PTSD will try to insulate themselves from the conditions that remind them of traumatic experiences (e.g., they will stop driving, will not return to work, or will avoid dating or having close interpersonal relationships); and people who have panic disorder with agoraphobia will take great care not to experience the situations that trigger their fear.

Because avoidance is rewarded with emotional relief, the avoidant behavior is more likely to occur again when the person is faced with the same or similar circumstances. For example, when a socially phobic person decides not to go to a party and feels immediate relief from anxiety, his avoidance is reinforced. The next time an invitation is received for a social event, the person will likely continue the pattern of avoidance as a way of controlling the anxiety associated with anticipated social scrutiny. Each time he avoids social situations, his phobic behavior and his dysfunctional cognitions about social performance are further reinforced, and his symptoms become more deeply entrenched.

Video Illustrations 1 and 2, which you viewed earlier in the book (see Chapter 2, "The Therapeutic Relationship: Collaborative Empiricism in Action"; Chapter 3, "Assessment and Formulation"; and Chapter 5, "Working With Automatic Thoughts"), show symptom assessment and cognitive restructuring interventions used in the treatment of Gina, a woman with panic symptoms, agoraphobia, and a fear of riding in elevators. Additional videos from the treatment of Gina are featured later in this chapter. Gina associated having panic attacks with any closed-in space or any place from which escape would be difficult. Elevators became one of the conditioned stimuli for her panic attacks. Gina circumvented her fear of elevators by taking the stairs and avoiding riding the elevator when possible. Because her therapist recognized that avoidance was perpetuating her fear, he encouraged her to use behavioral methods to expose herself to the feared situation.

Another example of the reinforcing power of avoidance is observed in obsessive-compulsive disorder (OCD). When obsessional thoughts occur in persons with OCD, compulsive rituals are often used to stop the thoughts. When the obsession is counteracted (and thus avoided) with the compulsive behavior, anxiety is reduced. Therefore, the compulsive act is reinforced as a coping strategy because it dampens or turns off the aversive obsessional thought. Because of the reinforcement, the next time the obsessions occur, the compulsive ritual is likely to be repeated.

In summary, the key features of the contributions of learning theory to the CBT model for anxiety disorders are 1) an initial (unconditioned) stimulus causes a fearful (unconditioned) response and is generalized to conditioned stimuli that in turn produce conditioned responses; 2) a pattern of avoidance of the feared stimuli serves to reinforce the patient's belief that he cannot face the object or cope with the situation; and 3) the pattern of avoidance must be broken for the patient to overcome the anxiety.

Studies of cognitive processes in anxiety disorders (see Chapter 1, "Basic Principles of Cognitive-Behavior Therapy") and the development of cognitive methods for anxiety have enriched this basic behavioral model in several important ways. First, a number of investigations have shown that the automatic thoughts of persons with anxiety are characterized by illogical reasoning (e.g., magnification of the risk in situations, minimization of estimates of the person's ability to cope, catastrophic predictions of deleterious effects of being in the situation). Second, a developmental perspective suggests that fearful cognitions may be shaped by many life experiences, including teachings of parents and other influential people, which help shape core beliefs about risk, danger, and one's ability to manage these exigencies. Finally, many anxiety disorders (especially cases of generalized anxiety disorder, panic disorder, and OCD) cannot be traced back to a single fearful stimulus that set off a pattern of conditioned stimuli and avoidance. Therefore, a more complex formulation—which may include the effects of learning experiences during growth and development, the impact of automatic thoughts and core beliefs, and other potential influences (e.g., the entire gamut of biopsychosocial factors as discussed in Chapter 3, "Assessment and Formulation")—is recommended for treating anxiety disorders with CBT. We focus here on describing the behavioral elements of the overall CBT model. Cognitive interventions for anxiety are detailed further in Chapter 1, "Basic Principles of Cognitive-Behavior Therapy"; Chapter 5, "Working With Automatic Thoughts"; and Chapter 8, "Modifying Schemas."

Overview of Behavioral Treatment Methods

Behavioral methods for anxiety are directed primarily at severing the link between 1) the CS or UCS and 2) the fear response (CR or UCR).

$$UCS/CS \xrightarrow{\quad X \quad} UCR/CR$$

In learning theory, this process is referred to as unpairing the stimulus and response. Avoidance reduces fear elicited by the CS in the short run but does not uncouple the connection between the UCS/CS and UCR/CR. To interrupt this connection, the avoidance must be replaced with a more adaptive behavior.

Breaking the Stimulus-Response Connection

The most commonly used general procedures for unpairing the UCS/CS and the UCR/CR are *reciprocal inhibition* and *exposure*. Reciprocal inhibition is defined as a process of reducing emotional arousal by helping the patient experience a positive or healthy emotion that counteracts a dysphoric response. The usual method of implementing reciprocal inhibition is to induce a state of deep relaxation of voluntary musculature, thereby producing a state of calm largely incompatible with intense anxiety or arousal. When a person becomes deeply relaxed in the presence of a feared stimulus, the stimulus and response can be unpaired. When this method is practiced regularly, the power of the stimulus to evoke fear and avoidance can fade or be eliminated.

Exposure uncouples the stimulus-response connection in a different way. As a coping strategy, exposure has the opposite effects of avoidance. If a person intentionally exposes himself to a stressful stimulus, he is likely to experience fear. However, fear is generally time limited because physiological arousal cannot be maintained at a heightened state indefinitely. Fatigue occurs, and in the absence of new sources of arousal, the person will begin to adapt to the situation. For example, if a person who is afraid of heights is taken to the top floor of a tall building and asked to look out the window, he will be frightened, even panicked. But eventually the fear response will be depleted and a normal homeostatic state will return. With repeated exposures, the physiological response to the feared situation should decrease as the person concludes that the stimulus can be faced and managed.

Cognitive restructuring techniques can aid the process of uncoupling a fearful response from a stressful stimulus by facilitating the relaxation response and by promoting involvement in exposure-based interventions. Methods that reduce or turn off negative thoughts can lower tension levels, thereby helping the person enjoy the physical and emotional sensations of relaxation. Thought stopping is a commonly used method to accomplish this goal. This technique does not require analysis of negative automatic thoughts as described in Chapter 5, "Working With Automatic Thoughts." Instead, a deliberate, conscious effort is made to replace fearful cognitions with more pleasant or calming thoughts, such as relaxing mental images.

Another cognitive restructuring method that can help in the unpairing of anxiety responses from their stimuli is decatastrophizing. Decatastrophizing helps the patient to 1) systematically evaluate the likelihood of an imagined catastrophic outcome occurring on exposure to the stimulus, 2) develop a plan to reduce the probability that such an outcome will occur, and 3) create a strategy to cope with the catastrophe should it occur. Procedures for thought stopping and decatastrophizing are described more fully later in this chapter (in the section "Step 3: Basic Skills Training").

Sequencing Behavioral Interventions for Anxiety Symptoms

The sequence of behavioral interventions is similar in the treatment of different types of anxiety disorders. First the therapist assesses symptoms, anxiety triggers, and existing coping strategies. Then specific targets of intervention are defined to guide the course of therapy. Next the patient is taught basic skills for coping with the thoughts, feelings, and behaviors that characterize the anxiety disorder. Finally, these skills are used to assist patients in systematically exposing themselves to anxiety-provoking situations.

Step 1: Assessment of Symptoms, Triggers, and Coping Strategies

In assessing anxiety disorders, it is important to clearly delineate 1) the events (or memories of events or streams of cognitions) that serve as triggers for the anxiety response; 2) the automatic thoughts, cognitive errors, and underlying schemas involved in the overreaction to the feared stimulus; 3) the emotional and physiological responses; and 4) habitual behaviors such as panic or avoidance symptoms. Thus all elements of the basic cognitive-behavioral model are evaluated and considered in developing the formulation and treatment plan. General assessment methods used in CBT are discussed in Chapter 3, "Assessment and Formulation." The major form of assessment is a careful interview targeted at uncovering the key symptoms, triggers for anxiety, and salient cognitions and behaviors (see Video Illustration 1).

Specialized diagnostic and rating measures also may be useful in the assessment phase of working with patients with anxiety disorders. The Structured Clinical Interview for DSM-IV-TR (First et al. 2002) can help clinicians make accurate diagnoses. In addition, self-report measures (e.g., the Beck Anxiety Inventory [Beck et al. 1988], the Fear of Negative Evaluation Scale [Watson and Friend 1969], and the State-Trait Anxiety Inventory [Spielberger et al. 1983]) and clinical rating scales (e.g., the Yale-Brown Obsessive Compulsive Scale [Goodman et al. 1989]) can be used to measure the severity of anxiety symptoms.

The thought record described in Chapter 4, "Structuring and Educating," can be a helpful tool for assessing anxiety-provoking situations because it provides a structure for documenting triggering events as well as automatic thoughts associated with those events. Identification of places, situations, and people that elicit anxiety will aid in preparation for exposure interventions. Spotting cognitive errors can give the therapist leads for possible cognitive restructuring interventions. Another useful strategy is to ask patients to make notes of things they encounter that cause anxiety and to rate the intensity of the reaction on a scale of 0–100, with 100 indicating the most extreme emotion. These types of ratings can be used for baseline assessments and for measuring progress in achieving treatment goals.

Assessment of the behavioral component of the anxiety response should go beyond identifying avoidance reactions to include a more detailed analysis of actions the patient takes to cope with the anxiety. For example, there may be healthy coping strategies that are being used (e.g., problem solving, employing a sense of humor, meditation) that could be strengthened or given more emphasis. However, patients with anxiety disorders frequently engage in *safety behaviors*—actions that may fall short of outright avoidance but still perpetuate the anxiety reaction. To illustrate, a person with social phobia may be able to force himself to go to occasional parties, but he copes with anxiety by going immediately to the buffet and gulping down more food than he would ordinarily eat, staying by his wife's side so that she can do all the talking, and going to the bathroom much more frequently than needed to get away from the crowd. Although he is attending the party, he is engaging in safety behaviors that are part of his pattern of avoidance. To be successful in overcoming problems such as the social anxiety experienced by this patient, the therapist will need to obtain a full picture of coping strategies, both maladaptive and adaptive, and design interventions that will help the patient identify all of the avoidant behaviors and expose himself to the full experience of facing and managing the feared situation.

One especially important type of safety behavior occurs when a patient has involved a family member or friend in helping her cope. Sometimes family support can be quite useful in overcoming anxiety, but there is a risk that the attempts of others to help can inadvertently reward or reinforce avoidant behavior and thus perpetuate the anxiety symptoms. For example, when Gina's panic attacks made her too fearful to drive a car or face crowds, her fiancé gave her assistance by driving her to work. Also, her friends went with her to the cafeteria or brought take-out food to her (see Video Illustration 1 and the formulation in Chapter 3, "Assessment and Formulation"). When a positive consequence follows a behavior, the behavior is likely to occur again. This phenomenon is called *positive reinforcement*. Although the efforts to help made by Gina's fiancé and friends were not intended as rewards, these efforts nonetheless served as positive reinforcements and may have played a role in the maintenance of her panic symptoms.

When you plan interventions for anxiety symptoms, you will need to take environmental contingencies into consideration. If the full range of reinforcers of anxiety are not considered, your efforts at helping the patient achieve more independence from fear could easily be thwarted by subtle safety behaviors that escape your notice or by a well-intentioned family member who facilitates avoidance as a coping strategy.

Step 2: Identifying Targets for Intervention

It is not unusual for an individual to have multiple manifestations of anxiety. Gina, the woman in the video illustrations, was fearful of driving, of riding in elevators, of being in crowds, of receiving social scrutiny, and of having additional panic attacks. As demonstrated in Video Illustrations 1 and 2, what often works best is to start by targeting a symptom or goal that is most easily accomplished, so that the patient can build confidence by having early success. Also, lessons learned from experiences in managing one feared situation can often be generalized to provide effective coping strategies for other anxieties.

When Dr. Wright asked Gina to prioritize her targets for overcoming anxiety, she decided to delay her worst fear, driving by herself, until she could make some headway in reducing anxiety about going to the cafeteria where she worked. Gina's fear of eating in a crowded cafeteria stemmed from an irrational notion that she would humiliate herself by dropping her tray of food, breaking the dishes, and causing people to stare at her and laugh. Although the problem with going to the cafeteria was modest in comparison with her anxiety about driving, it offered a good opportunity to learn basic CBT methods and to obtain a sense of accomplishment in using them.

Sometimes patients choose to start by tackling their most challenging problem because it is vitally important to them or because environmental pressures are forcing them to make progress quickly (e.g., anxiety about a job interview when the patient is unemployed and running out of money). If in your judgment the patient will need some further experience before being able to effectively address the situation, you can break the overall problem into pieces. In a manner similar to the graded task assignment approach described in Chapter 6, "Behavioral Methods I: Improving Energy, Completing Tasks, and Solving Problems," target a circumscribed part of the problem for immediate attention. Whether you begin by attacking the most difficult situation or you ease the patient into exposure therapy in a step-by-step fashion, the basic skills training described below can give patients tools to overcome their anxiety.

Step 3: Basic Skills Training

Several core CBT skills can help patients successfully engage in exposure-based interventions for anxiety disorders. We detail five of these methods below: relaxation training, thought stopping, distraction, decatastrophizing, and breathing retraining.

Relaxation Training

The goal of relaxation training is to help patients learn to achieve a relaxation response—a state of mental and physical calmness. Muscle relaxation is one of the principal mechanisms for achieving the relaxation response. Patients are taught to systematically release tension in muscle groups throughout the body. As muscular tension is decreased, the subjective feeling of anxiety is usually reduced. A common method for teaching patients deep muscle relaxation is to follow the steps outlined in Table 7–1. Some therapists also find it useful to read relaxation induction instructions to their patients or to ask them to listen to an audiotape of these instructions. Basco (in press) provides an example of a script for reading relaxation instructions to patients.

Learning Exercise 7–1. Relaxation Training

1. Try out the relaxation instructions in Table 7–1 on yourself. Work on achieving a state of deep muscle relaxation.

2. Then practice the induction procedure with one or more of your patients with anxiety symptoms.

Thought Stopping

As noted previously (see "Breaking the Stimulus-Response Connection" earlier in this chapter), thought stopping is different from most cognitive interventions in that it does not involve an analysis of negative thoughts. Its aim is to stop the process of negative thinking and replace it with more positive or adaptive thoughts. Thought stopping may be helpful for some patients with anxiety disorders such as phobias and panic disorder. However, studies of patients with OCD have shown an intensification of obsessions when the patient makes a conscious effort to suppress them (Abramowitz et al. 2003; Purdon 2004; Rassin and Diepstraten 2003; Tolin et al. 2002). Therefore, if thought stopping is not useful in helping the patient reduce worrisome thoughts, try another technique. Procedures for thought stopping are as follows:

1. *Recognize* that a dysfunctional thought process is active.
2. *Give a self-command to stop the thought*—for example, tell yourself in a commanding tone, "Stop!" or "Quit thinking that way!" The command can either be an internal thought or be spoken aloud.

Table 7–1. A method for relaxation training

---

1. *Explain the rationale for relaxation training.* Before beginning the relaxation induction, give the patient an overview of the reasons for using relaxation training. Also briefly explain the overall method.

2. *Teach patients to rate their level of muscle tension and anxiety.* Use a 0–100 scale, where a rating of 0 is equivalent to no tension or anxiety and 100 represents maximum tension or anxiety.

3. *Explore the range of muscle tension.* Because the focus of relaxation training is primarily on reducing muscular tension, it often helps to ask the patient to try to tighten one fist to the maximum level (100) and then let it completely relax to a rating of 0 or to the lowest level of tension he can achieve. Then the patient can be asked to try to tighten one hand to the maximum level while relaxing the other hand as much as possible. This exercise usually shows the patient that he can gain voluntary control over his state of muscle tension.

4. *Teach the patient methods for reducing muscle tension.* Starting with the hands, try to help the patient reach a state of full relaxation (rated as a 0 or close to 0). The primary methods used in cognitive-behavior therapy are a) exerting conscious control over muscle groups by monitoring tension and telling oneself to relax the muscles, b) stretching the targeted muscle groups through their full range of motion, c) gentle self-massage to soothe and relax tight muscles, and d) use of calming mental images.

5. *Help the patient systematically relax each of the major muscle groups of the body.* After the patient has achieved a state of deep relaxation of the hands, ask him to allow the relaxation to spread through the entire body, one muscle group at a time. A commonly used sequence is hands, forearms, upper arms, shoulders, neck, head, eyes, face, chest, back, abdomen, hips, upper legs, lower legs, feet, and toes. However, any sequence can be chosen that you and the patient believe will work best for him. During this phase of the induction, all of the methods from step 4 that have proved helpful can be repeated. We often find that stretching allows the patient to find especially tense muscle groups that may require extra attention.

6. *Suggest mental images that may assist in relaxation.* Mental images that you suggest (or that are evoked by the patient) can divert attention from worrisome thoughts and help him to concentrate on achieving the relaxation response. For example, the induction recommended by Basco (in press) contains instructions such as a) "Picture your shoulder muscles being tight like a wet dishrag that you are wringing. Let your shoulders loosen just as you would untwist the dishrag and shake it loose"; and b) "Let your tensions melt away and drip off your fingertips and onto the floor like ice melting slowly." Use a calm, soothing, and genuine vocal tone as you suggest these images.

7. *Ask the patient to practice the relaxation induction method regularly.* Usually it takes a considerable amount of practice before patients can master the deep relaxation technique. Therefore, it is often useful to suggest that patients perform relaxation exercises for homework assignments. When relaxation is part of the treatment plan for anxiety disorders, it is also important to check on the patient's progress in using this technique in subsequent sessions.

---

3. *Evoke a visual image* to reinforce the command, such as a stop sign, a red traffic light, or the gloved hand of a police officer directing traffic.
4. *Switch the image* from the stop sign to a pleasant or relaxing scene. The image should be something created in your mind such as a vacation memory, the face of a pleasant person, or a photograph or painting you have seen. The positive image can be amplified by deep muscle relaxation and by embellishing the image with details such as the time of day, weather conditions, and sounds associated with the image.

Each step should be rehearsed in session by asking the patient to first generate the upsetting thought(s) and then implement the thought-stopping strategies. Ask the patient for feedback on his experience, and then make any needed adjustments to the procedures. For example, if the positive image was difficult to create or sustain, choose another scene or modify the image to make it more vivid. Test the modified plan in the session before assigning its practice as homework.

Distraction

The imagery technique described in "Thought Stopping" above is a commonly used CBT distraction method. Imagery can also be used to augment other behavioral interventions, including breathing retraining (see Video Illustration 14). When using imagery, try to help the patient generate several positive, calming scenes that she can use to relax and, at least temporarily, defuse the intensity of anxiety-ridden thoughts. Myriad other possibilities exist for helping patients use distraction to lessen the impact of intrusive or worrisome thoughts. Commonly used distractions are reading, going to a movie, working on a hobby or craft project, socializing with friends, or spending time on the Internet. When distraction is employed, the therapist needs to be careful to monitor the activities so that they are not being used to avoid feared situations or to escape from the exposure-based methods described later in this chapter. Effective use of distraction should facilitate participation in exposure and other behavioral interventions by reducing the frequency or intensity of automatic thoughts and lowering physical tension and emotional distress. Some studies have suggested that distraction may be more useful than thought stopping for reducing obsessional thoughts in OCD (Abramowitz et al. 2003; Rassin and Diepstraten 2003).

Decatastrophizing

The general principles for using decatastrophizing methods are explained in Chapter 5, "Working With Automatic Thoughts," and are illustrated in

Video Illustration 2. This vignette shows Dr. Wright working with Gina to revise her automatic thoughts about the disasters that she predicts will happen if she faces the crowds in her cafeteria. If the techniques used in this illustration are not fresh in your memory, it might be useful to replay Video Illustration 2 to learn about cognitive restructuring methods for persons with anxiety disorders. Also, watching Video Illustration 2 may provide helpful background information for understanding the methods demonstrated in the other videos that accompany this chapter. Here are some procedures that you can use to help patients reduce their catastrophic predictions:

1. *Estimate the likelihood* that the catastrophic outcome will occur by asking patients to rate their belief on a scale from 0% (completely unlikely) to 100% (absolute) certainty. Note the answer for future outcome assessments.
2. *Evaluate the evidence* for and against the likelihood that a catastrophic event will occur. Monitor patients' use of cognitive errors, and use Socratic questions to help patients discriminate between fears and facts.
3. *Review the evidence list* and ask patients to reestimate the likelihood of the catastrophe occurring. Usually there should be a lowering of the original value from step 1. If the probability estimate increases (the worry becomes more believable), inquire about the pieces of evidence from step 2 that made the feared outcome seem more likely. Apply cognitive restructuring methods from Chapter 5, "Working With Automatic Thoughts," if necessary.
4. *Assess perceived control* by asking patients to rate the extent to which they believe they have control over the occurrence of the event or the outcome of the event. Use a scale of 0% (no control) to 100% (complete control). Make a note of this value for later review.
5. *Create an action plan* by brainstorming strategies to reduce the likelihood that the catastrophe will occur. Have the patient write down the actions she could take to improve on or prevent the feared outcome.
6. *Develop a plan for coping* with the catastrophe if it should occur.
7. *Reassess* the perceived likelihood of the catastrophic outcome, as well as the degree of perceived control over the ultimate outcome. Compare this assessment to the original ratings and discuss any differences.
8. *Debrief* by asking the patient what it was like to talk about his catastrophic thoughts in this way. Reinforce the value of decatastrophizing as part of the treatment plan.

Breathing Retraining

Breathing retraining is often used in the treatment of panic disorder because hyperventilation is a frequent symptom of panic attacks. The most frequently used strategy for breathing retraining for panic attacks begins with asking the patient to increase the respiration rate before reducing it. The patient may be instructed to breathe rapidly and deeply for a short time (maximum of a minute and a half) to replicate the respiration experience of a panic attack. The next step is to ask the patient to attempt to breathe slowly until regaining normal control over his respiration. Most patients with panic disorder report that this exercise closely approximates the feeling of a panic attack. Thus it is helpful to allay catastrophic fears about possible outcomes by explaining what is happening physiologically when a person hyperventilates.

Therapists can help patients learn to control their breathing by teaching methods for slowing respirations such as counting breaths, using the second hand of a watch to time breaths, and using positive imagery to calm anxious thoughts. Video Illustration 14 shows Dr. Wright simulating the hyperventilation that often occurs in panic attacks and asking Gina to do the same. Then they work on normalizing breathing patterns and using positive imagery to enhance the effects of controlling the rate of respiration.

> ▶ **Video Illustration 14.**   Breathing Retraining:
> Dr. Wright and Gina

Once mastered in session, breathing retraining exercises are recommended for use as homework. They should be rehearsed daily until confidence is gained in using the technique. Patients should also be instructed to attempt to use this method in anxiety-provoking situations, with the caveat that their expectation for control of anxiety should be tempered until the skill has been fully developed.

> **Learning Exercise 7–2.**   Breathing
> Retraining
>
> 1. After viewing Video Illustration 14, practice breathing retraining by role-playing with a colleague.
>
> 2. Rehearse overbreathing and then slowing the breathing rate to about 15 breaths per minute.
>
> 3. Practice using imagery to reduce anxiety and facilitate breathing retraining.

Step 4: Exposure

Exposure to anxiety-provoking stimuli is the final step in unpairing the stimulus-response connection in anxiety disorders. To counter the reinforcement cycle caused by avoidance, the patient is assisted in confronting stressful situations while using the cognitive restructuring and relaxation methods described above in "Step 3: Basic Skills Training." Although some anxiety symptoms such as simple phobias can be treated in a single session with *flooding* therapy (i.e., the patient is encouraged to directly face the feared stimulus while the therapist models coping with the situation), most exposure therapies use the *systematic desensitization* method. This procedure involves the development of a hierarchy of feared stimuli that is then used to organize a graded exposure protocol for overcoming anxiety a step at a time. The remainder of this chapter is devoted to providing details on the specific methods of exposure therapy and related techniques.

Developing a Hierarchy for Graded Exposure

The success of systematic desensitization, or graded exposure, often hinges on the quality of the hierarchy that is developed for this procedure. Some suggestions for developing effective hierarchies are noted in Table 7–2.

Video Illustration 15 shows Dr. Wright constructing a hierarchy for Gina to change her pattern of avoiding the cafeteria at work. She had been experiencing high levels of anxiety and panic attacks associated with her fear of being around others and embarrassing herself. During the session, Dr. Wright and Gina started to develop the hierarchy by generating seven items and observing that her level of anxiety was influenced by factors such as the time of day she went to the cafeteria, the number of people she encountered there, the type of dishes she used (i.e., paper or glass), and whether or not a friend accompanied her. After Gina and Dr. Wright listed the seven items and rated them for degree of anxiety, Dr. Wright asked Gina to complete a full hierarchy with 10–12 items as a homework assignment.

> ⏵ **Video Illustration 15.** Exposure Therapy—
> Constructing a Hierarchy: Dr. Wright and Gina

When you view the video, you will also note that Dr. Wright asked Gina if she could forecast an exposure activity that would be "over the top"—

Table 7–2. Tips for developing hierarchies for graded exposure

---

1. *Be specific.* Help the patient write out clear, definitive descriptions of the stimuli for each step in the hierarchy. Examples of overgeneralized or ill-defined steps are "Learn to drive again"; "Stop being afraid of going to parties"; and "Feel comfortable in crowds." Examples of specific, well-delineated steps are "Drive two blocks to the corner store at least three times a week"; "Spend 20 minutes at the neighborhood party before leaving"; and "Go to the mall for 10 minutes on a Sunday morning when there are very few people there." Specific steps will help both you and the patient make good decisions about the plan for progressing through the hierarchy.
2. *Rate the steps for degree of difficulty or amount of expected anxiety.* Use a scale of 0–100, with 100 representing the greatest difficulty or anxiety. These ratings will be used to select the steps for exposure at each session and to measure progress. The usual effect of progressing through a hierarchy is to have significant reductions in the ratings for degree of difficulty or anxiety as each step is mastered.
3. *Develop a hierarchy that has multiple steps of varying degrees of difficulty.* Coach the patient on listing a number of different steps (typically 8–12) that range in degree of difficulty from very low (ratings of 5–20) to very high (ratings of 80–100). Try to list steps throughout the entire range of difficulty. If the patient lists only steps with high ratings or can think of no midrange steps, you will need to assist him in developing a more gradual and comprehensive list.
4. *Choose steps collaboratively.* As with any other cognitive-behavior therapy assignment, work together with the patient as a team to select the order of steps for graded exposure therapy.

---

an activity that would cause so much anxiety that a rating of 100 on the current hierarchy would be too low to capture the intensity of the experience. After thinking for a moment, Gina replied that dropping her tray on purpose would be so anxiety provoking that she would need to rate it about 125 on a 0–100 scale. Dr. Wright had suggested earlier that she might consider confronting her worst fear in order to get better control of her anxiety (see Video Illustration 2). The strategy of asking patients to generate ideas for activities that would justify over-the-top anxiety ratings can have several benefits: 1) ratings for other items on the hierarchy may be revised downward and thus appear to be more manageable; 2) spotting activities that cause extreme fear may stimulate the patient to think of other, less anxiety-provoking items for the hierarchy; and 3) the over-the-top items can eventually be added to the list of exposure activities and thus help the patient to fully confront the feared stimuli.

Imaginal Exposure

There are two types of exposure, *imaginal exposure* and *in vivo exposure*. When imagery is used for graded exposure, the therapist asks the patient to try to immerse himself in the scene and to imagine how he might react. Cues are given to help the patient experience the anxiety-related stimuli as vividly as possible. The imaginal exposure technique was used in a therapy session to help Donald, a man who had developed PTSD after a car accident.

Case Example

Donald had extreme anxiety coupled with a total avoidance of driving. The therapist had worked with Donald to develop a full hierarchy for resuming normal driving, but Donald reported that he was not yet ready to put the hierarchy into action in real-life situations.

The first four steps in the hierarchy and their anxiety ratings were 1) start the car, back out of the garage, drive to the end of the driveway, and then return to the garage—10; 2) drive around the block early in the morning when there is not much traffic—20; 3) drive six blocks to the gas station and return home—35; 4) drive about 12 blocks, through two traffic signals, to the grocery store and then return home—40. Part of the dialogue from Donald's use of imaginal exposure is shown below.

Therapist: Which of the early steps would you like to walk through here in the treatment session?

Donald: Let's try the one about driving to the gas station.

Therapist: OK. Try to picture yourself getting into the car and leaving your driveway. What do you see, how are you feeling, what are you thinking?

Donald: I'm gripping the wheel so hard that my knuckles are turning white. I'm thinking, I can't handle this....I'll freak out....I'll lose control...or someone will barrel around the corner and run into me.

Therapist: Now try to check out the predictions. How accurate are they? What is the likelihood of all of those bad things happening?

Donald: There's a very low chance of anything like that happening. I'm just rattled because of the accident.

Therapist: What can you do to calm yourself and continue on your way to the gas station?

Donald: Breathe easy, tell myself to stop the scary thoughts, remind myself that I know how to drive and that the chances of another wreck are low.

Therapist: Can you keep driving? Can you pull out of the driveway?

Donald: Yes, I want to do it.

The therapist went on to help Donald use imagery to continue the trip to the gas station and also to expose himself to the fear associated with the next step—driving to the grocery store. Eventually Donald was able to use in vivo exposure to complete his recovery from PTSD triggered by a traumatic car accident.

Imaginal exposure can be particularly helpful in the treatment of PTSD, in which thoughts of the trauma are avoided and thereby retain their anxiety-provoking value. Imagery can also be beneficial in exposure therapy for OCD. Obsessional thoughts can be evoked in session and then quieted using relaxation or distraction. In addition, exposure and response prevention protocols for compulsions can be worked through first with imagery to help the patient gain skills and confidence in being able to stop these behaviors. You also might consider using imaginal exposure when triggering situations are difficult to replicate (e.g., simple phobias like fear of blood or fear of objects that may be encountered rarely).

Some of the major points to keep in mind when using imaginal exposure are the following: 1) use environmental cues to create vivid images of the feared stimuli; 2) use cognitive restructuring, relaxation, thought stopping, or other CBT methods to decrease anxiety and dispel the negative image; 3) present the images in a hierarchical fashion, asking the patient to take the lead in choosing the specific targets; 4) coach the patient on ways to cope with the anxiety; and 5) repeat the imaginal exposure until the anxiety is extinguished.

Because exposure therapy may be most effective if the patient can confront feared stimuli in real-life situations, it is also advisable to attempt to engage the patient in subsequent in vivo exposure whenever possible. The case illustration of treating Donald's anxiety involved use of imagery as a method of preparing him for exposure to real-life driving experiences. Other examples of using imagery to help patients make the transition to in vivo exposure include work with fear of flying (e.g., conducting imagery exercises in the office, followed by taking actual plane trips) and agoraphobia (e.g., practicing steps for going to a mall with imagery and then implementing the hierarchy in vivo).

In Vivo Exposure

In vivo exposure involves direct confrontation with the stimulus that arouses fear in the patient. Depending on the resources of your clinical environment, it may be possible to conduct in vivo exposure during therapy sessions. Fear of heights, elevators, and some social situations can be recreated, and the therapist can accompany the patient as she engages in the exposure experiences. There are advantages and disadvantages to the therapist being present during in vivo exposure. The positive features of this approach include the opportunity for the therapist to 1) model effective anxiety management techniques, 2) encourage patients to confront their fears, 3) provide timely psychoeducation, 4) modify catastrophic cognitions, and 5) give constructive feedback. However, accompaniment by the therapist can make a threatening situation seem safer, just as having a friend or family member along can reduce levels of anxiety. Therefore, caution should be exercised that the therapist's actions do not facilitate the pattern of avoidance. To complete the exposure process, more work will usually need to be done outside of sessions when the patient is unaccompanied.

Video Illustration 16 shows Dr. Wright helping Gina perform in vivo exposure for her fear of riding in elevators. He uses this opportunity to model ways of managing the situation and does on-the-spot cognitive restructuring to assist in the exposure process.

> ▶ **Video Illustration 16.**   In Vivo Exposure Therapy:
> Dr. Wright and Gina

Most applications of in vivo exposure are accomplished in homework assignments without the therapist being present. To implement this type of in vivo exposure effectively, you will need to engage the patient in a process of working through the hierarchy, beginning with exposure to stimuli that are rated low for degree of difficulty or anxiety and building toward the most threatening scenario. The patient should assess his level of anxiety before and after the exposure exercise and should keep a record of the amount of anxiety reduction achieved. Each subsequent trial should aim at reducing anxiety a little more, until the situation no longer elicits fear. To add to the value of this intervention, ask the patient to make a prediction about how threatening the exposure will be and how well he anticipates being able to handle it. Frame the exposure as an experiment to test these predictions.

After assigning in vivo exposure as a homework assignment, you will need to debrief the patient at the next session. Ask her to compare her predictions to the actual outcome. If the situation was less threatening and was handled better than anticipated, ask what she thinks this means for future efforts at coping with her anxiety. If the patient found that the situation was more difficult than anticipated or that she handled it more poorly than planned, make the next step easier to accomplish or review the methods used to control fear. If there were difficulties in applying coping strategies, practice them in session. If unanticipated obstacles made the situation more complex, try to help the patient find a way to surmount these problems.

Response Prevention

Response prevention is a general term for methods used to help patients stop behaviors that are perpetuating their disorder. In CBT for anxiety disorders, exposure and response prevention are typically used together. Patients are encouraged to expose themselves to feared situations while agreeing *not* to follow through with their usual avoidance response. For example, response prevention interventions in the treatment of OCD can be as simple as leaving the room where a compulsive ritual takes place (e.g., walking away from the sink after washing the hands once) or agreeing to participate in an alternative behavior. For checking behaviors around the house, the person can agree to leave his home after the first round of checks and not return home for a specified period despite feeling the urge to do so. Response prevention methods usually work best if they are determined collaboratively, instead of being a prescription from the therapist. The patient and therapist decide together on specific goals for response prevention, and then the patient logs his efforts to follow the plan.

Rewards

Positive reinforcement increases the odds that the rewarded behavior will occur again. Thus, in constructing exposure protocols it may be helpful to consider the role of positive reinforcement in encouraging adaptive behaviors such as approaching feared situations. Family members and friends can praise the patient and provide rewards or incentives for accomplishing exposure goals. For example, they might go out to dinner with the patient to celebrate achieving an important milestone in the exposure process. Patients can also reward themselves for their accomplishments in combating fears. Rewards can be anything patients find pleasant or positive. The size of the reward should match the perceived size of the accomplishment. Smaller rewards such as food (e.g., eating a favorite ice cream) might be used for taking beginning or intermediate steps to face fears. Larger rewards (e.g., buying something special, taking a trip) could be planned for overcoming bigger hurdles.

Pacing Exposure Therapy

Research studies on CBT for panic disorder, social phobia, and uncomplicated OCD have shown substantial reductions in symptoms with relatively brief treatment protocols (i.e., 12–16 sessions; Barlow et al. 2000; Clark 1997; Foa et al. 2005). However, the number of sessions required for effective treatment can range from a single visit for simple phobias to lengthy protocols for persons with refractory OCD (Öst et al. 2001; Salkovskis 2000). In making decisions on the speed of exposure therapy, take into account the diagnosis, the presence or absence of comorbid conditions (e.g., other anxiety disorders, depression, substance abuse, personality disorders), patient strengths such as intelligence and resilience, the patient's motivation and readiness for change, and the patient's responses to beginning efforts to follow exposure protocols.

Some patients will quickly grasp the exposure concept and will push themselves to undertake challenges. Gina, for example, was able to productively engage in a rapid exposure paradigm. If patients are responding favorably to the first parts of the exposure protocol, they can be encouraged to press ahead. However, other patients may have more embedded, difficult-to-treat problems with anxiety (e.g., contamination fear or hoarding behavior in OCD) that will slow progress in working through an exposure hierarchy. In implementing exposure protocols, therapists need to pace interventions at a rate that does not push patients beyond their capacity to change but instead challenges and inspires them to break patterns of avoidance and conquer their fears.

Learning Exercise 7–3.   Exposure Therapy

1. Ask a colleague to role-play a patient with an anxiety disorder, or do this exercise with one of your patients.

2. Using the tips in Table 7–2, write out a hierarchy for exposure to a specific feared situation.

3. Identify at least eight separate steps, ranging from low to high degrees of difficulty.

4. Choose a beginning target for exposure therapy.

5. Use imaginal exposure to help prepare the person for in vivo exposure.

6. Try to spot potential problems in carrying out the plans for exposure, and coach the person in methods of overcoming these difficulties.

7. Keep practicing exposure therapy methods until you master this key behavioral technique.

Summary

Cognitive-behavioral methods for anxiety disorders are based on the concept that persons with these conditions develop unrealistic fears of objects or situations, respond to feared stimuli with excessive anxiety or physiological activation, and then avoid triggering stimuli to escape from the unpleasant emotional reaction. Each time patients avoid an anxiety-provoking situation, they collect further evidence that they can't cope or manage. But if the pattern of avoidance can be interrupted, they can learn that the situation can be tolerated or mastered.

The behavioral interventions described in this chapter are directed primarily at stopping avoidance. Patients are taught how to reduce emotional arousal, how to moderate dysfunctional cognitions that amplify anxiety, and how to systematically expose themselves to feared situations.

A four-step process is used as a general template for behavioral interventions for anxiety disorders: 1) assessment of symptoms, triggers for anxiety, and coping methods; 2) identification and prioritization of targets for therapy; 3) coaching in basic skills for managing anxiety; and 4) exposure to stressful stimuli until the fear response is significantly reduced or eliminated. These methods are first practiced in therapy sessions and then are applied in homework assignments to extend treatment gains into the patient's daily life.

References

Abramowitz JS, Whiteside S, Kalsy SA, et al: Thought control strategies in obsessive-compulsive disorder: a replication and extension. Behav Res Ther 41:529–540, 2003

Barlow DH, Gorman JM, Shear MK, et al: Cognitive-behavioral therapy, imipramine, or their combination for panic disorder: a randomized controlled trial. JAMA 283:2529–2536, 2000

Basco MR: The Bipolar Workbook: Tools for Controlling Your Mood Swings. New York, Guilford, in press

Beck AT, Epstein N, Brown G, et al: An inventory for measuring clinical anxiety: psychometric properties. J Consult Clin Psychol 56:893–897, 1988

Clark DM: Panic disorder and social phobia, in Science and Practice of Cognitive Behaviour Therapy. Edited by Clark DM, Fairburn CG. New York, Oxford University Press, 1997, pp 121–153

First MB, Spitzer RL, Gibbon M, et al: Structured Clinical Interview for DSM-IV-TR Axis I Disorders, Research Version, Patient Edition (SCID-I/P). New York, Biometrics Research, New York State Psychiatric Institute, 2002

Foa EB, Liebowitz MR, Kozak MJ, et al: Randomized, placebo-controlled trial of exposure and ritual prevention, clomipramine, and their combination in the treatment of obsessive-compulsive disorder. Am J Psychiatry 162:151–161, 2005

Goodman WK, Price LH, Rasmussen SA, et al: The Yale-Brown Obsessive Compulsive Scale, I: development, use, and reliability. Arch Gen Psychiatry 46:1006–1011, 1989

Öst LG, Alm T, Brandberg M, et al: One vs five sessions of exposure and five sessions of cognitive therapy in the treatment of claustrophobia. Behav Res Ther 39:167–183, 2001

Purdon C: Empirical investigations of thought suppression in OCD. J Behav Ther Exp Psychiatry 35:121–136, 2004

Rassin E, Diepstraten P: How to suppress obsessive thoughts. Behav Res Ther 41:97–103, 2003

Salkovskis PM, Richards C, Forrester E: Psychological treatment of refractory obsessive-compulsive disorder and related problems, in Obsessive-Compulsive Disorder: Contemporary Issues in Treatment (Personality and Clinical Psychology Series). Edited by Goodman WK, Rudorfer MV. Mahwah, NJ, Lawrence Earlbaum Associates, Inc, 2000, pp. 201-221

Spielberger C, Gorsuch R, Lushene R, et al: Manual for the State-Trait Anxiety Inventory. Palo Alto, CA, Consulting Psychologists Press, 1983

Tolin DF, Abramowitz JS, Przeworski A, et al: Thought suppression in obsessive-compulsive disorder. Behav Res Ther 40:1255–1274, 2002

Watson D, Friend R: Measurement of social-evaluative anxiety. J Consult Clin Psychol 33:448–457, 1969

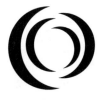

8

Modifying Schemas

When you help people change schemas, you will be working at the bedrock of their self-concept and way of living in the world. Schemas are the core beliefs that contain fundamental rules for information processing. They provide templates for 1) screening and filtering information from the environment, 2) making decisions, and 3) driving characteristic patterns of behavior. The development of schemas is shaped by interactions with parents, teachers, peers, and other significant people in the person's life, in addition to life events, traumas, successes, and other formative influences. Genetics also play a role in the production of schemas, by contributing to temperament, intellect, special skills or lack of skills (e.g., athletic prowess, body shape, attractiveness, musical talent, problem-solving ability), and biological vulnerability to both mental and physical illnesses.

There are several reasons why it is important to understand your patient's underlying schemas. First, a basic theory of cognitive-behavior therapy (CBT)—the stress-diathesis hypothesis—specifies that maladaptive core beliefs, which may lie under the surface and have relatively few negative effects during periods of normality, can be primed by stressful events to become potent controllers of thinking and behavior during ill-

---

Items mentioned in this chapter that are available in Appendix 1, "Worksheets and Checklists," are also available as a free download in larger format on the American Psychiatric Publishing Web site: http://www.appi.org/pdf/wright.

ness episodes (Clark et al. 1999). Thus, efforts to revise dysfunctional schemas may have positive benefits in two principal domains: 1) relief of current symptoms and 2) improved resistance to stressors in the future. CBT has been shown to have strong effects in reducing the risk for relapse (Evans et al. 1992; Jarrett et al. 2001). Although the exact mechanisms for this feature of CBT are not known, it is presumed that schema modification may be involved.

Another reason for focusing treatment interventions on core beliefs is that patients typically have a mix of different types of schemas. Even patients with the most severe symptoms or profound despair have adaptive schemas that can help them cope. Although maladaptive schemas may seem to be in full charge during an illness episode, efforts to uncover and strengthen positively oriented beliefs can be quite productive. Therefore, it is important to explore and burnish the adaptive parts of patients' basic cognitive structures.

The cognitive-behavioral theory of personality, as articulated by Beck and Freeman (1990), specifies that self-concept, character types, and habitual behavioral patterns can be best understood by examining core beliefs. For example, a person with obsessive-compulsive personality traits might have deeply held schemas such as "I must be in control" and "If you want something done right, do it yourself." It is likely that this person would have a behavioral repertoire (e.g., rigidity, tendency to be controlling toward others, difficulty delegating authority) consistent with these beliefs. Another person who has a cluster of dependency-related schemas (e.g., "I need others to survive"; "I'm weak...I can't make it on my own") might cling to others and lack assertiveness in interpersonal relationships. In contrast, a more adaptive group of schemas—such as "I can figure things out"; "I can handle stress"; "I like challenges"—would be associated with effective behaviors for problem solving.

CBT for Axis I disorders is typically geared toward symptom relief instead of personality change. Nevertheless, an analysis of the core beliefs and compensatory behavioral strategies that contribute to the patient's personality makeup can help you build an in-depth formulation and help you design treatment interventions that take full account of the patient's vulnerabilities and strengths. In addition, some patients with Axis I disorders may have treatment goals that include elements of personal growth. They may want to become more flexible, break patterns of excessive dependency, or overcome long-standing problems with self-esteem. In such cases, the treatment process can be enriched by articulating and revising schemas that may block the way to achieving these goals. In Chapter 10, "Treating Chronic, Severe, or Complex Disorders," we briefly outline some recommended modifications of CBT for treatment of personality disturbances. If you are interested in learning more about CBT for Axis II disorders, we recommend the excellent books by Beck and Freeman (1990) and by Linehan (1993). Our primary emphasis here is on helping you learn how to identify schemas in patients with Axis I conditions and how to use CBT to modify these core beliefs (Table 8–1).

Table 8–1. Methods for identifying schemas

Using various questioning techniques
Performing psychoeducation
Spotting patterns of automatic thoughts
Conducting a life history review
Using schema inventories
Keeping a personal schema list

Identifying Schemas

Using Questioning Techniques

Guided discovery, imagery, role play, and other questioning techniques used for automatic thoughts also are used to uncover schemas. However, several different questioning strategies are used when working on the schema level of cognitive processing compared with work on automatic thoughts. Because schemas may not be readily apparent to the patient or may not be revealed by standard questioning, a hypothesis should be developed about what core beliefs might be present. Then the therapist can frame questions that point in the direction of the presumed schemas. This type of guided discovery is illustrated in the case example below.

Case Example

Allison was a 19-year-old woman with depression and bulimia who had been hospitalized after a suicide attempt.

Therapist: What was going through your mind before you took the overdose?
Allison: That I couldn't keep going. Life was just too much for me. I couldn't please anyone. I felt like a failure.
Therapist: That must have been really hard for you…to think that you couldn't please anyone and that you were a failure. What was going on in your life that made you think these things were true?
Allison: I've messed up everything. No matter how hard I try, I can never satisfy my parents—or anyone else. They want me to date the per-

fect guy, and I always seem to come up with losers. Maybe if I was a size 4 instead of a size 12, everything would be OK.

Although the therapist could have started to work immediately on Allison's beliefs that she couldn't please others and that she was a failure, the therapist decided to continue to use guided discovery to search for an underlying schema about perfectionism. The therapist's case formulation at this point included a hypothesis that Allison's depression, suicidality, and bulimia were being influenced to a large extent by a core belief that she had to do things perfectly to gain approval or to achieve success.

> *Therapist:* It sounds like you have to reach high standards to feel good about yourself. I wonder if you have a basic rule in your mind about what you have to do to be loved or to be a success.
> *Allison:* I know that I'm never happy unless I get things just right. When I was growing up, I always had to get the best grades....Straight A's were always expected. And my mother kept putting me on a diet. I'll bet I was the only third grader in the city who had to count calories.
> *Therapist:* It must have been tough to meet all those expectations. From what you've told me about your current situation, it looks like you are still struggling with trying to be the best. I mentioned something about a basic rule a moment ago. I have a hunch that you developed a fundamental belief about the way you need to act to gain the approval of your parents or of any other important people in your life. What do you think that rule might be?
> *Allison:* I must be perfect. If I'm not perfect, I won't be accepted.

In this example of guided discovery, the therapist had a fairly easy task of helping Allison articulate a core belief that was having a strong effect on her behavior. Often the questioning process will take longer or will need to go through multiple paths before reaching an important schema. Mood shifts can be good clues that a consequential schema is at work. These sudden displays of intense feelings can serve as excellent entry points for a series of questions directed at uncovering a core belief. Another one of Allison's schemas was identified via a mood shift coupled with an imagery exercise.

> *Therapist:* How are you adjusting to being in the hospital?
> *Allison:* Everybody has been nice. I like most of the nurses. (*Appears calm and mildly happy.*) But I can't stand it when they bring out the dinner cart. Why do they have all of that food? (*Mood becomes much more anxious.*)
> *Therapist:* I noticed that you got pretty nervous when you talked about the food cart. What upsets you about the way they serve meals here?

Allison: Everybody eats so much food, and the server just piles it on. I can't stop myself if I get in that food line.
Therapist: Can you imagine yourself lined up to get served at the food cart? Try to picture yourself standing in line. What thoughts are going through your mind?
Allison: I'll eat everything on the cart; I'll totally lose control.
Therapist: How much control do you think you have over your behavior?
Allison: I have no control.

One of the most popular CBT methods for uncovering schemas, the *downward arrow technique,* involves a series of questions that reveal increasingly deeper levels of thinking. The first questions are typically directed at automatic thoughts. However, the therapist infers that an underlying schema is present and constructs a chain of linked questions that build on a supposition (to be tested and modified later) that the patient's cognitions are providing an accurate representation of her true self. Most of the questions follow this general format: "If this thought that you have about yourself is true, what does it mean about you?"

Because the downward arrow technique requires the patient to assume (for the purposes of the intervention) that negative or hurtful cognitions are actually true, this method should not be attempted before a good therapeutic relationship has been established and there have been previous therapy successes in modifying maladaptive cognitions. The patient should be fully aware that the purpose of the questioning is to bring out core beliefs that will probably need to be changed, and that the therapist is not trying to convince her of the validity of troubling schemas. A kind and empathic tone of questioning, and sometimes a light touch of hyperbole or judicious humor, can help make the downward arrow technique work to best effect.

The video illustration of Dr. Thase uncovering Ed's schema shows how to use this technique effectively. Ed was introduced in Chapter 3, "Assessment and Formulation," where a case formulation for his treatment was developed. Illustrations from this case were also featured in Chapter 4, "Structuring and Educating" (section on "Psychoeducation") and Chapter 6, "Behavioral Methods I: Improving Energy, Completing Tasks, and Solving Problems" (sections on "Activity Scheduling" and "Graded Task Assignments"). When you view Video Illustration 17, note how Dr. Thase initiates the intervention by identifying some of Ed's automatic thoughts about the breakup of an important relationship. Dr. Thase and Ed have previously done work on modifying automatic thoughts, so Ed knows that spotting a maladaptive cognition can be an important step in gaining relief from symptoms. A highly collaborative and empirical therapy style is evident throughout the vignette. Several of the key questions and Ed's responses are diagrammed in Figure 8–1.

Ed: (Describes his automatic thoughts about breaking up with his wife)
I messed that up....I'll never get it right....I'll never be with somebody.

Dr. Thase: *What if that were true?*

Ed: *I'm going to mess everything up. I'm just not capable of getting this intimate relationship thing right.*

Dr. Thase: *And if that were true?*

Ed: *I'm no good....I'm worthless....I'm defective.*

Dr. Thase: *And if that happened to be true, what would that mean about your future?*

Ed: *I'll never be able to do anything right. I'll end up by myself.*

Figure 8–1.   The downward arrow technique.

▶ **Video Illustration 17.**   The Downward Arrow Technique: Dr. Thase and Ed

It may take a fair amount of practice before you become proficient at using the downward arrow technique. Building your knowledge of commonly held schemas in Axis I disorders and in personality types can help you formulate directions for questioning. Gaining experience in knowing when to exert pressure to go further and when to back off will help you to be more effective in using inference chaining methods. It is important to keep the emotional tone at a plane that is conducive to learning and that is experienced as helpful by the patient. Yet the process of uncovering maladaptive schemas often generates painful affects.

Experienced cognitive-behavior therapists who use the downward arrow technique try to pitch the questions at just the right level to assist the patient in revealing an important core belief—and to make the questioning process a highly therapeutic experience. We recommend that you practice the learning exercises for uncovering schemas and that you review the list of tips for using the downward arrow technique that are presented in Table 8–2.

Table 8–2. How to use the downward arrow technique

---

1. Start the questioning by targeting an automatic thought or a stream of cognitions that is causing distress. Choose an automatic thought that is likely to be driven by a significant underlying schema.
2. Generate a hypothesis about a possible schema or set of schemas that may underlie this automatic thought.
3. Explain the downward arrow technique so that the patient understands your intent in asking these difficult questions.
4. Be sure that you and the patient are fully collaborating in using this technique. Emphasize the collaborative empirical nature of cognitive-behavior therapy (CBT).
5. Anticipate timing and pacing concerns in advance. Ask yourself questions such as "Is this a good time to attempt to uncover this schema?" "Is the patient ready to come to grips with this core belief?" "How fast and how intensively should I ask questions that will lead the patient's thinking to this schema?" and "What signs would tell me to go slower or to end this line of questioning?"
6. Think ahead to what you will do after the schema is identified. What positive benefits will there be to revealing this schema? What will be the next steps after the core belief comes out? How will you help the patient make good use of knowing about this schema?
7. Use if-then questions that progressively reveal deeper levels of cognitive processing. For example, "I've heard you mention several times that you have trouble making friends. If it's true that you have trouble making friends, what does this tell us about the way that others may see you? How about the way you view yourself?"
8. Be supportive and empathic as core beliefs are uncovered. Convey an attitude that knowing about schemas will help the patient build self-esteem and learn to better cope with problems. Even if a negatively toned core belief is partially accurate, CBT can be directed at acquiring skills for tempering the maladaptive schema and its behavioral consequences.

Learning Exercise 8–1. Questioning Methods for Core Beliefs

1. Practice guided discovery for uncovering schemas by asking yourself a series of questions that start with one of your own situation-specific automatic thoughts and then reveal deeper levels of cognition. Try out the downward arrow technique on yourself. Use this method to get in touch with one or more of your personal schemas. If possible, try to uncover a schema that has some maladaptive effects, in addition to a schema that is largely

positive or adaptive. Write down the questions
and your answers in your notebook.

2. Next, enlist a classmate or helper to role-play
   guided discovery and the downward arrow
   technique for identifying core beliefs, or
   practice these methods with patients you have
   in treatment.

3. Make a list of the strengths and weaknesses
   that you have in asking questions to uncover
   core beliefs. What are you doing well? What
   do you need to practice more intensively? Are
   you able to develop an accurate formulation in
   a timely manner? Can you phrase questions in
   a manner that instills hope while still getting
   to painful and troubling core beliefs? Are you
   paying enough attention to recognizing
   adaptive schemas? Identify any problems you
   are having in implementing questioning
   strategies for schemas, and discuss possible
   solutions with classmates, colleagues, or
   supervisors.

Educating Patients About Schemas

Psychoeducation about schemas is typically implemented concurrently
with the questioning methods described above in "Using Questioning
Techniques." In addition to brief explanations in therapy sessions, we often
recommend readings or other educational experiences to help patients
learn about and identify their schemas. *Mind Over Mood* (Greenberger and
Padesky 1996) contains exercises directed at teaching patients how to recognize their assumptions and core beliefs. *Getting Your Life Back* (Wright
and Basco 2001) includes examples of both adaptive and maladaptive
schemas that can help patients recognize their own basic rules of information processing.

The computer program *Good Days Ahead* (Wright et al. 2004) has a
number of interactive scenarios designed to promote the discovery and
modification of schemas. Computer-assisted CBT can be especially helpful in teaching patients about core beliefs because it uses stimulating
multimedia learning experiences that can point the way to cognitions
that may not be apparent on the surface. Also, computer-assisted CBT
employs learning enhancement techniques that promote rehearsal and
recall. In a controlled study of computer-assisted CBT versus standard

CBT, it was found that patients who utilized the *Good Days Ahead* computer program had greater improvement in scores on the Dysfunctional Attitude Scale (a measure of core beliefs; Beck et al. 1991) than those who received standard CBT (Wright et al. 2005).

Spotting Patterns of Automatic Thoughts

If recurrent themes can be recognized in automatic thoughts, this often indicates that a core belief is behind these clusters of more superficial, situation-specific cognitions. There are several good methods for finding schemas in patterns of automatic thoughts.

1. *Recognize a theme during a therapy session.* When using guided discovery or other questioning methods, listen for themes that play over and over. Exploring such themes can frequently lead to key schemas. For example, this pattern of automatic thoughts—"Jim doesn't respect me....My children never listen to me....It doesn't matter what I do at work, they'll always treat me like I hardly exist"—might be stimulated by core beliefs such as "I'm a nothing" or "I don't deserve respect."

2. *Review thought records in a therapy session.* Thought records can be treasure troves for material that will help you find schemas. Compare several thought records that have been completed on different days to see if there are any recurrent patterns of automatic thoughts. Ask the patient to see if she can recognize consistent themes. Then use guided discovery or the downward arrow technique to uncover related core beliefs.

3. *Assign review of thought records for a homework assignment.* After examining a thought record in a treatment session and explaining the process of spotting schemas, ask the patient to look over additional records between sessions and to record any core beliefs that she can recognize. Such homework assignments can have many benefits, including a) identification of schemas that might not be apparent during a therapy session, b) increased awareness of the powerful effects of core beliefs, and c) acquisition of self-help skills for uncovering schemas.

4. *Review a written list (or a computer-generated inventory) of automatic thoughts.* If the patient has completed an automatic thoughts questionnaire or has recorded a comprehensive list of her common automatic thoughts, it may be useful to check over this inventory to see if any clusters of thoughts may be linked to core beliefs. Consider using this alternative procedure if you are having trouble identifying schemas through guided discovery and other questioning methods. Viewing a large number of automatic thoughts may help you and the patient spot beliefs that otherwise would have gone unrecognized.

We present a learning exercise here that you can use to practice finding underlying schemas in patterns of automatic thoughts. You can also use this exercise to help your patients gain skills in recognizing their core beliefs.

> **Learning Exercise 8–2.** Finding Schemas in Patterns of Automatic Thoughts
>
> Instructions: Match one number to each of the letters in the exercise.

Automatic Thoughts	Maladaptive Schemas
1. "You'll lose everything.... You'll be out on the street.... It's only a matter of time before things will fall apart."	____ A. I'm a fake.
	____ B. Without a man, I'm nothing.
	____ C. I'm not as good as other people.
2. "This job is too much for me....I don't know what I'm doing....Everyone is bound to find out soon."	____ D. No matter how hard I try, I'm bound to fail.
3. "Ruth is calling me just because I'm lonely and miserable....My husband didn't want me....Why would anyone want to be around me?"	
4. "Everyone else seems so intelligent and has so much to say. Compared to them, I'm a real loser."	

Answers: A: 2; B: 3; C: 4; D: 1.

Source.   Adapted with permission of The Free Press, a Division of Simon & Schuster Adult Publishing Group. From *Getting Your Life Back: The Complete Guide to Recovery From Depression* by Jesse H. Wright M.D., and Monica Ramirez Basco, Ph.D. Copyright © 2001 by Jesse Wright and Monica Ramirez Basco. All rights reserved.

Conducting a Life History Review

Because schemas are shaped by life experiences, one valuable method of uncovering these basic rules is to ask the patient to go back in time to remember formative influences that may have promoted the development of either maladaptive or adaptive beliefs. This type of retrospective review can be accomplished through guided discovery, role play, and homework assignments. As with other methods of identifying schemas, an in-depth formulation can help point you in directions that will yield results. Instead of doing a global review of developmental history, try to focus on interpersonal relationships, events, or circumstances that have previously been shown to be hot topics. For example, if your patient has already told you that he never felt comfortable around his peers and shied away from social experiences, you might focus your inquiries on especially memorable social interchanges from childhood or adolescence. Your goal with this line of questioning would be to elicit schemas about personal competence and acceptance by others.

Traumatic events, troubled relationships, or perceived physical or personality defects can be obvious targets for historical reviews of schema formation. However, it is important not to forget positive influences that may have promoted the development of adaptive beliefs. The following types of questions can be used to assist patients in getting in touch with life experiences that have played a role in schema development.

1. *Ask about influential people:* "Which people have made the biggest difference in your life?" "Besides your family, are there any teachers, coaches, friends, classmates, or spiritual leaders who have influenced the way you think?" "How about people who have given you trouble or have put you down?" "Which people have boosted your confidence or given you encouragement?"

2. *Ask about core beliefs that may have been shaped by these experiences:* "What negative messages did you get about yourself from all of the arguments with your family?" "How did your parents' divorce affect your self-esteem?" "What affirmative beliefs came out of your successes in school?" "What did you learn about yourself by going through the divorce and getting away from the abusive relationship?"

3. *Ask about interests, jobs, spiritual practices, sports, and other activities that are important to the patient:* "In what way have your interests and abilities in music changed how you see yourself?" "What core beliefs do you have about your work skills?" "How has your view of yourself been influenced by your spiritual beliefs?" "How about involvement in artistic pursuits, travel, or hobbies—could these activities have affected your self-concept?"

4. *Ask about cultural and social influences:* "What impact has your cultural background had on the way you see the world?" "How has growing up as a minority affected your self-concept?" "What beliefs might have been influenced by living in a small town your entire life and being so close to family and friends?"

5. *Ask about education, readings, and self-study:* "How did your time in school influence your basic beliefs?" "Which books have you read that you think might have changed the way you think about yourself?" "What ideas did you develop from reading that book?" "Can you remember any other learning opportunities that have made a difference in your attitudes about life?"

6. *Ask about the possibility of transforming experiences:* "Have you had any life-shaping experiences that you haven't told me about?" "Could there have been an event that opened your eyes to a whole new way of seeing the world?" "What attitudes or beliefs came out of that experience?"

Using Schema Inventories

Inventories of commonly held core beliefs are another useful technique for helping patients identify their schemas. These instruments include the Dysfunctional Attitude Scale (Beck et al. 1991), a lengthy questionnaire primarily used in research; and another highly detailed scale, the Young Schema Questionnaire (Young and Brown 2001; Young et al. 2003). A briefer inventory of schemas was developed for the computer program *Good Days Ahead* (Wright et al. 2004). We provide this schema checklist in Learning Exercise 8–3 and in Appendix 1, "Worksheets and Checklists," so that you will have this tool available for clinical practice.

Schema inventories can be useful when patients are having difficulty recognizing their core beliefs. Seeing a variety of possible schemas can stimulate their thinking and can help them recognize beliefs that may be causing trouble or could be reinforced to build self-esteem. Taking a schema inventory is especially useful in generating a list of adaptive beliefs. In our experience in supervising trainees, we often find that insufficient attention is paid to identifying positive rules of thinking. Administering a schema inventory guarantees that you will spend some time scanning the patient's belief system for points of strength and for opportunities for growth.

Even when patients seem to readily identify their underlying core beliefs through guided discovery and other questioning techniques, administering a schema inventory can add depth to your formulation. We typically find that patients endorse both negative and positive schemas that we had not identified previously. In addition, discussion of reactions to completing a schema inventory can lead to discovery of other valuable information about core beliefs. Sometimes an underlying schema is not listed in the inventory, but the beliefs that are included trigger a series of thoughts that reveal one of the patient's most important underlying assumptions.

For the next learning exercise, we would like you to take this schema inventory adapted from some of our earlier work. Because the list was designed to be used for people with significant depression or anxiety, many of the dysfunctional schemas are expressed in absolute terms. However, our clinical experience and research with the inventory indicates that patients frequently endorse the maladaptive schemas on this list (Wright and Basco 2001). We recommend that you start to administer a schema inventory to the patients you are treating with CBT and that you discuss the responses in your therapy sessions.

Learning Exercise 8–3. Taking an Inventory of Your Schemas

Instructions: Use this checklist to search for possible underlying rules of thinking. Place a check mark beside each schema that you think you may have.

Healthy Schemas	Dysfunctional Schemas
___ No matter what happens, I can manage somehow.	___ I must be perfect to be accepted.
___ If I work hard at something, I can master it.	___ If I choose to do something, I must succeed.
___ I'm a survivor.	___ I'm stupid.
___ Others trust me.	___ Without a woman (man), I'm nothing.
___ I'm a solid person.	___ I'm a fake.
___ People respect me.	___ Never show weakness.
___ They can knock me down, but they can't knock me out.	___ I'm unlovable.
___ I care about other people.	___ If I make one mistake, I'll lose everything.
___ If I prepare in advance, I usually do better.	___ I'll never be comfortable around others.
___ I deserve to be respected.	___ I can never finish anything.
___ I like to be challenged.	___ No matter what I do, I won't succeed.
___ There's not much that can scare me.	___ The world is too frightening for me.
___ I'm intelligent.	___ Others can't be trusted.
___ I can figure things out.	___ I must always be in control.
___ I'm friendly.	___ I'm unattractive.
___ I can handle stress.	___ Never show your emotions.
___ The tougher the problem, the tougher I become.	___ Other people will take advantage of me.
___ I can learn from my mistakes and be a better person.	___ I'm lazy.
___ I'm a good spouse (and/or parent, child, friend, lover).	___ If people really knew me, they wouldn't like me.
___ Everything will work out all right.	___ To be accepted, I must always please others.

Source. Adapted with permission from Wright JH, Wright AS, Beck AT: *Good Days Ahead: The Multimedia Program for Cognitive Therapy.* Louisville, KY, Mindstreet, 2004.

Keeping a Personal Schema List

We've made the point many times in this book that writing down material learned in therapy sessions and in homework assignments can be a critical step in being able to recall and effectively use CBT concepts. When you are working with core beliefs, it is especially important to emphasize the value of keeping a written record and regularly reviewing these notes. Because schemas are often latent or below the surface of everyday thinking, awareness of core attitudes may erode quickly if not reinforced. In our clinical practices we have seen many situations where we have worked hard to identify a key schema in a therapy session, yet with the pressure of current environmental events and the passage of time, patients seem to "forget" about this core belief unless we draw their attention to it.

A customized schema list can be an excellent method of recording, storing, and reinforcing the knowledge that you and the patient have gained about core adaptive and maladaptive beliefs. In the opening phase of work on schemas, there may be only a few entries on this list. But as therapy proceeds, more schemas will be added, and maladaptive core beliefs will be modified with techniques described in the next section, "Modifying Schemas." Thus the personal schema list is a fluid entity that should show steady evidence of improvement throughout the course of CBT.

> **Learning Exercise 8–4.** Developing a
> Personal Schema List
>
> 1. Use the methods described in this chapter to develop your own personal schema list. Try to write down as many adaptive and maladaptive schemas as possible.
>
> 2. Practice developing personal schema lists with one or more of your patients. Review the lists regularly in therapy sessions. Edit and modify the lists as progress is made to change schemas.

Modifying Schemas

After you have helped your patient identify underlying schemas, you can begin to work on changing dysfunctional basic rules of thinking and behaving. When you are doing this, it is wise to remember that schemas are often deeply embedded and have been practiced and reinforced for many

---

Table 8–3. Methods for changing schemas

Conducting Socratic questioning
Examining the evidence
Listing advantages and disadvantages
Using the cognitive continuum
Generating alternatives
Performing cognitive and behavioral rehearsal

---

years. Therefore, it is unlikely that patients will change them dramatically by gaining insight alone. To modify these key operational principles, patients typically need to go through a concentrated process of examining the beliefs, generating plausible alternatives, and rehearsing the revised schema in real-life situations (Table 8–3).

Socratic Questioning

Good Socratic questions can often help patients see inconsistencies in their core beliefs, appreciate the impact of schemas on emotions and behavior, and begin the process of change. One of the principal goals of Socratic questioning is to stimulate a sense of inquiry, thus moving the patient away from a fixed, maladaptive view of self and the world to a more inquisitive, flexible, and growth-promoting cognitive style. Here are some suggestions for asking Socratic questions that may help patients be more open to revising their core beliefs.

1. *Develop a formulation to direct your line of questioning.* Have a good idea where you are heading. Chess masters plan many moves ahead and have a variety of strategies in mind to react to the possible actions of the other player. Act like a great chess player in planning ahead. Of course, your Socratic questions will be collaborative instead of competitive.

2. *Use questions to help patients see contradictions in their thinking.* Patients typically have a variety of core beliefs, some of which give them competing messages. In a classic videotape, Aaron T. Beck (1977) asked a patient who was facing a divorce to explain the contradiction between her belief that she could not live without her husband and another belief that she had been happier and healthier before she got married. These types of questions can lead to rapid breakthroughs in understanding and a willingness to engage in subsequent action plans to change.

3. *Ask questions that encourage the patient to recognize adaptive beliefs.* In general, it is more likely that adaptive beliefs will be fully endorsed,

remembered, and acted on if the patient does a good deal of the work in uncovering positively toned schemas. Instead of telling patients that they have healthy attitudes or strengths to be used in fighting their problems, try to ask Socratic questions that get them highly involved in articulating adaptive core beliefs.

4. *Avoid asking leading questions.* Even if you have a good plan of what you would like the patient to see or do, don't ask questions in a manner that conveys that you already know the answers. Maintain the collaborative and empirical style of CBT. Remain open to following the train of the patient's thinking.

5. *Remember that questions that activate significant emotion may enhance learning.* If you can ask Socratic questions that either stimulate emotional arousal or sharply reduce emotional pain, the learning experience may be more meaningful and memorable for the patient.

6. *Ask questions that serve as a springboard for implementing other methods of changing schemas.* Good Socratic questions often prepare the way for other more specific methods of modifying core beliefs. Think of Socratic questions as keys that can unlock doors to learning. After you ask an effective Socratic question, be prepared to implement other methods such as examining the evidence, generating alternative beliefs, or using the cognitive continuum, all described in the next sections.

Examining the Evidence

In Chapter 5, "Working With Automatic Thoughts," we explain how to examine the evidence for automatic thoughts. The procedures for examining the evidence for schemas are very similar. However, because maladaptive core beliefs are so long-standing and have often been reinforced by actual negative outcomes, criticism, dysfunctional relationships, or traumas, the patient may be able to generate considerable evidence that the belief is true. A man who believes that he is a loser may have had many instances of negative outcomes such as job losses, marital breakups, or financial problems. A woman who tells you that she is unlovable may recount a number of rejections by men. Therefore, when examining the evidence for schemas, you may need to acknowledge that problems have existed and to be empathic with the patient's life travails.

Even when patients produce plausible evidence that dysfunctional beliefs have some degree of validity, there are often numerous opportunities for helping these individuals reinterpret the meaning of negative outcomes, find counterbalancing evidence against the belief, and work on modifying behaviors to have more success in the future. Dr. Thase shows

Schema I want to change: I'm defective.

Evidence for this schema:	Evidence against this schema:
1. I messed up my job.	1. I've maintained a decent job. I've received journalism awards.
2. I've had a failed marriage.	2. My marriage went well for a while. My wife liked a lot of the things I did.
3. I always felt that "my shoes are going to fall off; I'm toast."	3. I haven't lost everything.
4. I've had problems at school and in athletics.	4. I lettered in track in college.
5. My family was a mess; I always felt that "I'm one of them."	5. I have a positive relationship with my daughter.

Cognitive errors: Magnifying, ignoring the evidence, overgeneralizing.

Modified schema: I'm a person with some strengths and some weaknesses. I can get through rough times.

Figure 8–2. Worksheet for examining the evidence for schemas: Ed's example.

how to do this in Video Illustration 18. Ed's exercise for examining the evidence is presented in Figure 8–2.

> ▶ **Video Illustration 18.** Examining the Evidence for Schemas: Dr. Thase and Ed

As Dr. Thase demonstrates in the video illustration, examining the evidence can be a powerful agent for change. When you implement the method of examining the evidence with your own patients, keep in mind the suggestions listed in Table 8–4.

The treatment of Allison, the 19-year-old woman with bulimia and depression described earlier in "Using Questioning Techniques," illustrates how an intervention to examine the evidence led to a productive homework assignment with specific behavioral goals. At this point in the treatment process, Allison's depression had improved and she was no longer suicidal. She had been discharged from the hospital and was continuing with outpatient CBT. Her therapist helped her develop a worksheet for the schema "I must be perfect to be accepted" (Figure 8–3). Note that Allison generated a fair amount of evidence against the statement and also added several observations about her cognitive errors. However, it appeared that she still needed more work on developing an alternative core belief. The blank worksheet for examining the evidence for schemas is available in Appendix 1, "Worksheets and Checklists," so that you can make copies to use with your patients.

Table 8–4.   How to examine the evidence for schemas

---

1. Briefly explain the procedure before beginning to examine the evidence.
2. Use an empirical approach. Engage the patient in a process of taking an honest look at the validity of the schema.
3. Write out the evidence on a worksheet. The first time through this procedure, it may work best for you to write down the evidence. Shift responsibility for writing to the patient whenever possible.
4. Worksheets can be initiated in therapy sessions and then completed for homework assignments, thus getting the patient fully involved in the process of generating and recording evidence.
5. Often evidence for schemas is absolutistic and is supported by cognitive errors and other dysfunctional information processing. Help the patient spot these errors in reasoning.
6. Where there is evidence that patients have had recurring problems with relationships, acceptance, competence, social skills, or other key functions, use this information to design intervention strategies. For example, a person with negative core beliefs about social competence may be helped by behavioral methods that break patterns of avoidance and teach skills needed to be facile in social settings.
7. Be creative in generating evidence against maladaptive core beliefs. Ask Socratic questions that stimulate different ways of viewing the situation. Because patients can have a fixed, negative view of themselves, your energy and imagination may be needed to help them find reasons to change.
8. Collect as much evidence as possible against dysfunctional schemas. This information will help patients refute core beliefs and will also provide important openings for other cognitive-behavior therapy interventions.
9. Use the method of examining the evidence as a platform for helping the patient make specific modifications in core beliefs. After examining the evidence with the patient, ask him or her to think about possible changes that will lead to healthier rules of thinking. Write these ideas down on the worksheet for examining the evidence, and follow up with other interventions described in this chapter.
10. Develop a homework assignment to build on the success of the exercise for examining the evidence. Possibilities might include adding more evidence to the worksheet, spotting cognitive errors, thinking of alternative schemas, or suggesting a behavioral assignment to practice acting in a new way that is consistent with the modified belief.

Listing Advantages and Disadvantages

Some maladaptive schemas are maintained through the years because they have a payoff. Even though the schema may be loaded with negative effects, it may also have benefits that induce the person to keep thinking and acting in the same dysfunctional way. Allison's schema, "I must be perfect to be accepted," is a good example of this type of core belief. Her

Schema I want to change: I must be perfect to be accepted.

Evidence for this schema:

1. My parents always pressured me to be the best at everything I do.

2. Men want thin women who look perfect.

3. When I got top grades in school, I won a scholarship. Everybody said I was a great student.

4. You need to excel to be popular. Who wants to be friends with somebody who is just average?

Evidence against this schema:

1. Even though my parents have high standards, I think they would accept me if I'm less than perfect. They aren't perfect themselves. I still love them, despite all of their flaws.

2. I have some friends who are overweight who have excellent relationships with their boyfriends.

3. Some of the happiest people I know aren't obsessed with perfectionism.

4. Other people who aren't perfect seem to be accepted for who they are. Maybe some people would be more comfortable having a relationship with a person who isn't perfect.

Cognitive errors in the "Evidence for" column: All-or-nothing thinking, magnifying, ignoring the evidence.

1. My parents have actually shown lots of caring and acceptance when I mess up or don't reach my goals. I know they would like me to be less obsessed about my weight.

2. There is a lot more to me than my weight or how flat my stomach is. I need to accept my other strengths.

3. Actually, I might make more friends if I didn't try so hard to be perfect. Setting such high standards may turn people off.

Now that I've examined the evidence, my degree of belief in the schema is: 30%.

Ideas I have for modifications to this schema:

1. I can strive for excellence but still accept myself when I don't reach perfection.

2. I will be happier and feel more accepted if I'm more realistic about reaching my goals.

Actions I will take now to change my schema and act in a healthier way:

1. I will write out a list of ways in which I am imperfect but am still a good person who deserves to be accepted.

2. I will purposely try to de-emphasize perfectionism in how I exercise by a) giving myself a day off at least twice a week and b) not counting or recording each repetition of work at the gym.

3. I will reduce perfectionism in my study habits by a) no longer logging the minutes I spend on each assignment, b) taking breaks from studying at least three times a week to do fun things (such as going to a movie or just goofing off with some friends), and c) changing my focus in study from always thinking about getting a perfect grade to enjoying the learning experience.

Figure 8–3. Worksheet for examining the evidence for schemas: Allison's example.

drive for perfectionism had made her miserable, but she had also had some major successes that were derived in part from her perfectionistic behavior. These double-sided schemas are very common, even in persons without any psychiatric symptoms. Perhaps you have some beliefs that have both advantages and disadvantages. Can you spot any of these schemas on your personal list?

> **Learning Exercise 8–5.** Finding Schemas
> With Advantages and Disadvantages
>
> 1. Review your personal list of schemas from Learning Exercise 8–4.
>
> 2. Identify a schema that may have served you well but that also may have a downside. Perhaps a schema has influenced you to work hard but has also caused tension or has taken a toll on your social life. No one has a complete set of fully adaptive schemas, so try to find one that has had both positive and negative effects.
>
> 3. List the advantages and disadvantages for this core belief.

Clinical application of the technique of listing advantages and disadvantages involves many of the same kinds of steps used for examining the evidence. First, you should briefly explain the procedure so the patient will know where you are heading. Then ask a series of questions geared toward developing a written record of advantages and disadvantages. Next, use this analysis to consider modifications that will make the schema more adaptive and less of a burden. Finally, design and implement a homework assignment to practice new behaviors.

Comparing advantages and disadvantages of a schema has several potential benefits. The full spectrum of effects of the schema can be seen, and exploring these different effects may stimulate creative ideas for change. Of course, listing the deleterious effects of the schema can highlight the downside of continuing to hold the belief. But it is just as important to know about the advantages of the schema. Patients are unlikely to give up maladaptive schemas and associated behaviors that give them substantial positive reinforcement unless these advantages are also provided by the modified belief.

Schema I want to change: I must be perfect to be accepted.

Advantages of this schema:	Disadvantages of this schema:
1. I have always been at the top of my class in school.	1. Perfectionism exhausts me.
2. I've stayed thin.	2. I have an eating disorder.
3. I worked very hard to learn to play the violin and was named to the state orchestra.	3. The only way I can feel happy is if everything is going just right.
4. Many of my classmates looked up to me.	4. Trying to be perfect distances me from others. They probably don't like me so much because it seems like I am trying to be better than them.
5. I got a scholarship to go to college.	5. I'm never really satisfied with myself. I think that I'm never good enough.
6. I've never gotten into trouble, other than having psychiatric treatment.	6. I can't relax and have fun. I get depressed a lot. I'm always tense and usually unhappy.

Ideas I have for modifications to this schema:

1. I can choose my targets for trying to do my best. For example, I can continue to study hard and have goals for a successful career. But I can back off in other areas of my life.
2. I can develop interests and hobbies where I don't have to be the best and can still enjoy doing things.
3. I can relax around friends and family and hope that they will accept me without my having to accomplish so much or be a perfect person.
4. I am more likely to be accepted by others if I try to be successful but don't go overboard in a relentless pursuit of perfection.

Figure 8–4. Worksheet for listing advantages and disadvantages: Allison's example.

When we try to generate alternative schemas, we often suggest that patients think of changes that will eliminate or greatly reduce the negative effects of the previous schema while holding on to at least some of the benefits. Allison's schema about perfectionism was a logical target for this type of intervention. Listing advantages and disadvantages led to several good ideas for revisions in her core belief (Figure 8–4).

The Cognitive Continuum

When schemas are expressed in absolute terms, patients may see themselves in an extremely negative light (e.g., "I'm a loser"; "I'm unlovable"; "I'm stupid"). If these types of schemas are present, the cognitive continuum technique can be used to help patients place their beliefs in a broader context and moderate their thinking.

Case Example

Jake, a man who viewed himself as a failure, was asked to construct a scale of 0–100 in which 100 equaled the greatest failure of all time, 50 equaled a moderate degree of being a failure, and 0 represented no failure at all during a lifetime. When Jake was first invited to rate himself, he put a mark of about 95 on this scale. At least he didn't rank himself as the greatest failure of all time. But he was probably still exaggerating the degree of his disappointments in life. The therapist used the following questions to help the patient modify his belief.

Therapist: You rated yourself as a 95 on the failure scale. Can you think of some examples of people who have been terrific failures, people who have totally messed up their lives in every way imaginable? These people have been a total failure in everything they did through their entire lives.

Jake: Well, it's hard to think of anybody who was a total failure in everything they ever did.

Therapist: There must be some examples of really colossal failures—people whom anyone would view as having absolutely no redeeming value.

Jake: Maybe it would be someone who never even finished the first grade, who couldn't be trusted to do anything right, who lied all the time, and who wasted his entire life doing drugs and getting drunk. He lost custody of all of his kids because he abused them and their mother. Even his own mother couldn't stand him and stopped speaking to him by the time he was 12. (*Jake chuckles a bit as he describes this hypothetical person.*)

Therapist: Now you're rolling. Could there be anyone worse than this?

Jake: Yes, I suppose someone who does bad things on purpose and ends up being a failure. I read about some of those high-flying executives who misled their companies, spent money like madmen, and then got caught. They deserve to go to jail.

Therapist: I'll bet you could think of some other examples of people who may be high on the failure scale, but let's take a look at the other end of the rankings. Can you think of anyone who never had a failure? Anyone who had everything work out perfectly in life? Anyone who never made a mistake or had a disappointment?

Jake: I suppose that nobody deserves to be ranked as being perfect, unless it's some big shot like a president or somebody like that.

Therapist: As long as you brought up the example of a big shot or a president, can you point out any flaws or failures of some of these types of people?

Jake: Sure, they are human just like everyone else. I remember reading about Winston Churchill. He was one of the greatest leaders of all time, but he got thrown out of office and went through a pretty bad depression. And how about Bill Clinton? He had his problems, didn't he?

Therapist: OK, I think you are getting the idea. Let's take a look at the scale again. When you consider all of the successes you have had in life and balance them against the difficult experiences, how would you rate yourself now?

Jake: I've had some failures. Losing my job was a big blow, and I always thought that I wasn't as good as most of my friends. But I'm not nearly as bad as somebody at the top of the scale. I guess I'd rate myself about 65.

Therapist: How would you like to view yourself?

Jake: Maybe somewhere between 25 and 35. That would be where I would put a lot of my friends.

Therapist: Could we make that one of the goals for our therapy: to build your self-esteem to the point where you believe you have more strengths than weaknesses?

Jake: Yes, I'd like to do that.

Generating Alternatives

Methods for changing core beliefs (e.g., Socratic questioning, examining the evidence, and listing advantages and disadvantages) described in this chapter often stimulate patients to consider alternative schemas. These key interventions can be very productive tools to help patients consider possible modifications in their basic rules of thinking. You can also adapt the techniques for finding rational alternatives to automatic thoughts (see Chapter 5, "Working With Automatic Thoughts") in your work with core beliefs. For example, you can encourage your patients to open their minds to a wide variety of possibilities by thinking like scientists or detectives—or to imagine that they are coaches who are building their strengths by helping spot positive but rational alternatives. The brainstorming method detailed in Chapter 5 can be particularly useful in generating alternatives to deeply held schemas. When we use this technique for revising core beliefs, we ask patients to try to step away from their old way of thinking and to consider a full range of potential changes.

Another way to help patients generate alternatives is to put a spotlight on the language of schemas. Consider, for example, the wording of these core beliefs: "I'm worthless"; "I'm no good at sports"; or "I will always be rejected." Pointing out the absolute terms in schemas and asking patients to consider using words that are less extreme is one way of generating healthier beliefs (e.g., "I've experienced rejections, but some family members and friends have stuck by me"). You can also help patients target if-then statements for change (e.g., "If people really knew me, they would know that I'm a fraud"; "If I don't meet all of his demands, he will leave me"; "If you get close to someone, they will always hurt you"). Educating people on the restricting nature of rigid if-then beliefs can prompt them to develop more flexible basic rules (e.g., "Getting close to someone has risks, but it doesn't always mean that I will get hurt"). Another technique that you might consider is to ask the patient to examine the wording of a core belief that may be offering some advantages but is having overall deleterious effects. Perhaps just changing one or two words will help the person to fine-tune the schema to a point where it is more adaptive or less damaging (e.g., revising "I must be in control" to "I like to be in control").

Some patients can productively use study, self-reflection, cultural activities, classes, and other growth-oriented experiences to explore possible changes in core beliefs. Readings might include inspirational, philosophical, or historical books that challenge the status quo of their thinking. Spiritual activities, theatrical or musical performances, the visual arts, stimulating public lectures, or adventures in the outdoors can provide opportunities for seeing the self and the world in different ways. These types of experiences may be especially useful for persons who are searching for a deeper sense of meaning or purpose in life. A few of the books that our patients have found most helpful include Victor Frankl's *Man's Search for Meaning* (1992), Jon Kabat-Zinn's *Full Catastrophe Living* (1990), Bernie Siegel's *Love, Medicine, and Miracles* (1990), and T. Byrum Karasu's *The Art of Serenity* (2003).

Cognitive and Behavioral Rehearsal

The three most important words in predicting success in changing schemas are *practice, practice,* and *practice.* Because insight alone is rarely enough to reverse entrenched core beliefs, you will need to devise strategies to help your patients try out revised schemas in real-world situations, learn from their achievements and roadblocks, and build skills for acting differently. Typically, rehearsal of possible modifications of schemas begins in therapy sessions and then extends via homework assignments into daily life. We discuss basic methods for cognitive and behavioral rehearsal in Chapter 5, "Working With Automatic Thoughts," and Chapter 6, "Behavioral Methods I: Improving Energy, Completing Tasks, and Solving Problems." To refresh your memory of how to perform rehearsal methods and to illustrate the use of this technique for schema change, we draw an example from Dr. Thase's treatment of Ed.

Previous video illustrations have shown Dr. Thase helping Ed develop alternatives to a core belief, "I'm defective." In the next vignette, he works with Ed to put a healthier schema into action. Although Ed has identified a weakness in his communication style with his daughter, he is also able to recognize that he has many strengths as a father and has the capacity to learn to be a more effective parent. Ed and Dr. Thase identify a specific

---

Table 8–5. Tips for practicing new schemas

---

1. Develop a written plan for trying out a new or revised schema. This plan should list the modified core belief in addition to specific behaviors that will be undertaken to put the revised schema into action.
2. Use imagery to rehearse the plan in a therapy session. Identify automatic thoughts, other schemas, or dysfunctional behavioral patterns that may interfere with the plan for change.
3. Develop coping strategies for overcoming obstacles.
4. Write out the amended plan on a coping card.
5. Develop a homework assignment to practice the new core belief and the adaptive behaviors in a specific real-life situation.
6. Coach the patient on ways to make the homework a productive experience.
7. Review the outcome of the homework in the next session, and make adjustments in the plan as necessary.
8. Keep the "practice, practice, practice" strategy in mind as you continue to help the patient modify schemas. Choose multiple targets for applying the principles for changing schemas.

---

communication problem and then practice ways of improving the relationship.

▶ **Video Illustration 19.** Rehearsing a Modified Schema: Dr. Thase and Ed

Many helpful strategies are available for practicing revised schemas. As shown in Video Illustration 19, Dr. Thase used imagery to help Ed generate ideas for change. Other commonly used methods include role-playing, brainstorming, and making coping cards. Presented in Table 8–5 are some suggestions for rehearsing modified schemas and behavioral plans for implementing these beliefs.

Growth-Oriented CBT

Although the goals of schema change are most commonly focused on symptom relief and relapse prevention, therapy can also be taken to another plane: working on personal meaning and growth. Even when patients are primarily concerned with relief of symptoms, it may be useful to look for core beliefs that may expand their potential for personal growth or may help them develop a full sense of purpose in life. Here are some examples of questions you might ask to find out if your patients have goals that may lead therapy in a growth-oriented direction: "When you get over the depression, will you still have some things you would like to work on in therapy?" "Do you have any additional goals for how your life might change after you retire (or your children leave home, or you get over the divorce, etc.)?" "You mentioned that you want to stop being a workaholic....What goals would you have for your life if you weren't working most of the time?"

Allison, the young woman with depression and bulimia, was so fixated on her pursuit of perfection and her struggle to maintain control that she was missing out on many of the potentially meaningful things in her world. However, when her symptoms began to subside, she was able to gain a richer perspective of the path ahead. Adaptive beliefs that had been obscured by her dysfunctional schemas could now be nurtured and strengthened (e.g., "I am a good friend"; "I would like to make a difference—to do something in my life that helps others"; "I love to be in nature, to appreciate the things around me").

The process of building growth-oriented schemas sometimes involves exploration of new terrain. Perhaps the patient has always thought that something was missing in his life, or that his life has not been centered on purposeful or meaningful things. Or perhaps a major loss has shaken his core values and constructs. In these types of situations, CBT can be directed toward helping the person grapple with existential questions and attempt to find ways to move beyond a loss, unlock potential, or commit to fresh ideas. In our book written for the general public, *Getting Your Life Back* (Wright and Basco 2001), we suggest several practical ways of searching for meaning. These ideas, largely drawn from the work of Victor Frankl (1992), can be assigned as self-help exercises for persons interested in building their sense of purpose or deepening their commitment to core values.

Some authors of articles and books on growth-oriented CBT have used the term *constructivism* or *constructivist cognitive therapy* to describe an approach in which the therapist helps the patient develop adaptive schemas that *construct* a new personal existence (Guidano and Liotti 1985; Mahoney 1995; Neimeyer 1993). The ultimate expression of constructivist cognitive therapy would be a treatment process in which a person is transformed to a higher level of personal authenticity and well-being. In our experience with CBT, such major transformations are uncommon. However, when persons continue in therapy beyond the symptom relief stage and work on reaching growth-oriented goals, the result can be very gratifying for both patient and therapist.

A full description of CBT methods for growth-oriented and constructivist cognitive therapy is beyond the scope of this basic text. However, we recommend that you consider dimensions of personal growth and meaning in developing formulations for treatment and that you devote at least a portion of the therapy effort to helping patients find adaptive core beliefs that can provide guidance for their future.

Learning Exercise 8–6. Modifying Schemas

1. Use a role-play exercise with a helper to examine the evidence for a schema and weigh its advantages and disadvantages.

2. Next use the techniques for generating alternatives described in this chapter.

3. Work out a plan for putting a modified schema into action. Include details on how the person will both think and act differently.

4. Then implement these methods for changing schemas in your work with patients.

5. Elicit at least one adaptive, growth-oriented schema from a patient, and develop a plan for putting this belief into action.

Summary

Changing core beliefs can be a challenging task. However, therapeutic work on modifying schemas can lead to important gains in self-esteem and behavioral effectiveness. Because schemas are deeply embedded basic rules of thinking, the therapist may need to show ingenuity and persistence in bringing them to the surface. Some of the commonly used methods for uncovering core beliefs are Socratic questioning, spotting schemas in patterns of automatic thoughts, and the downward arrow technique. Keeping a written list of schemas can help the therapist and patient remain focused on the change process.

To loosen the grip of maladaptive schemas, CBT methods encourage patients to step back from their core beliefs and check them for accuracy. Techniques such as examining the evidence and listing advantages and disadvantages can promote a broader perspective and stimulate the development of new schemas. When potential revisions in core beliefs are generated in therapy sessions or in homework assignments, a specific plan should be designed for trying out the schema in real-life situations. Repeated practice is usually required to cement modified schemas and to replace older, maladaptive rules of thinking. For some patients, a growth-oriented phase of CBT can help them work on adaptive core beliefs that add depth to their self-concept and enhance their sense of well-being.

References

Beck AT: Demonstration of the Cognitive Therapy of Depression: Interview #1 (Patient With a Family Problem) (videotape). Bala Cynwyd, PA, Beck Institute for Cognitive Therapy and Research, 1977

Beck AT, Freeman A: Cognitive Therapy of Personality Disorders. New York, Guilford, 1990

Beck AT, Brown G, Steer RA, et al: Factor analysis of the Dysfunctional Attitudes Scale in a clinical population. Psychol Assess 3:478–483, 1991

Clark DA, Beck AT, Alford BA: Scientific Foundations of Cognitive Theory and Therapy of Depression. New York, Wiley, 1999

Evans MD, Hollon SD, DeRubeis RJ, et al: Differential relapse following cognitive therapy and pharmacotherapy for depression. Arch Gen Psychiatry 49:802–808, 1992

Frankl VE: Man's Search for Meaning: An Introduction to Logotherapy. Boston, MA, Beacon Press, 1992

Greenberger D, Padesky CA: Mind Over Mood: Change How You Feel by Changing the Way You Think. New York, Guilford, 1996

Guidano VF, Liotti G: A constructivist foundation for cognitive therapy, in Cognition and Psychotherapy. Edited by Mahoney MJ, Freeman A. New York, Plenum, 1985, pp 101–142

Jarrett RB, Kraft D, Doyle J, et al: Preventing recurrent depression using cognitive therapy with and without a continuation phase: a randomized clinical trial. Arch Gen Psychiatry 58:381–388, 2001

Kabat-Zinn J: Full Catastrophe Living: Using the Wisdom of Your Body and Mind to Face Stress, Pain, and Illness. New York, Hyperion, 1990

Karasu TB: The Art of Serenity: The Path to a Joyful Life in the Best and Worst of Times. New York, Simon & Schuster, 2003

Linehan MM: Cognitive-Behavioral Treatment of Borderline Personality Disorder. New York, Guilford, 1993

Mahoney MJ (ed): Cognitive and Constructive Psychotherapies: Theory, Research, and Practice. New York, Springer, 1995

Neimeyer RA: Constructivism and the cognitive psychotherapies: some conceptual and strategic contrasts. Journal of Cognitive Psychotherapy 7:159–171, 1993

Siegel BS: Love, Medicine, and Miracles: Lessons Learned About Self-Healing From a Surgeon's Experience With Exceptional Patients. New York, HarperPerennial, 1990

Wright JH, Basco MR: Getting Your Life Back: The Complete Guide to Recovery From Depression. New York, Free Press, 2001

Wright JH, Wright AS, Beck AT: Good Days Ahead: The Multimedia Program for Cognitive Therapy. Louisville, KY, Mindstreet, 2004

Wright JH, Wright AS, Albano AM, et al: Computer-assisted cognitive therapy for depression: maintaining efficacy while reducing therapist time. Am J Psychiatry 162:1158–1164, 2005

Young JE, Brown G: Young Schema Questionnaire: Special Edition. New York, Schema Therapy Institute, 2001

Young JE, Klosko JS, Weishaar ME: Schema Therapy: A Practitioner's Guide. New York, Guilford, 2003

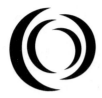

9

Common Problems and Pitfalls

Learning From the Challenges of Therapy

One of the advantages of the therapeutic approaches covered in this book is that their implementation is fairly straightforward. However, complications along the way can prevent the therapist from delivering interventions as intended. In Chapter 2, "The Therapeutic Relationship: Collaborative Empiricism in Action," we detail ways of managing problems in the therapeutic relationship (e.g., transference and countertransference). In this chapter, we describe some other common challenges that might be encountered in the delivery of cognitive-behavior therapy (CBT), suggest strategies for preventing each problem, and outline methods for responding when difficulties occur. These possible solutions are only a few of the many ways that cognitive-behavior therapists can surmount treatment obstacles. We encourage you to be creative and try out some of your own ideas for coping with treatment problems and pitfalls.

Homework Noncompletion

There can be many reasons why patients do not complete homework assignments. Possibilities include 1) problems with the therapist's technique (e.g., not preparing the patient well for the assignment; suggesting an assignment that is too challenging, too easy, or not useful); and 2) patient factors such as forgetfulness, low energy, lack of motivation, poor concentration, or negative attitudes about homework. There are several things you can do to avoid problems with homework or to cope effectively when homework is not completed as planned.

Prevention

1. *Request the patient's input when designing homework.* There are some standard homework assignments (e.g., reading about basic principles, completing thought records) that are used with most patients. However, many homework assignments can be tailor-made to meet the needs of the individual. When patients contribute to the design of homework assignments, they may be more likely to complete them. Specific homework tasks should be suggested by the patient as often as possible. The therapist should help shape the assignment in ways that maximize its chances for success.
2. *Rehearse homework assignments in advance.* If you demonstrate how to carry out a homework assignment by practicing at least a part of it in a therapy session, the patient may be more likely to understand the method and be able to implement it between sessions. It may also be useful to employ cognitive and behavioral rehearsal to help prepare the patient to implement a self-help method in real-world situations. A few examples of homework exercises that might be rehearsed first in a therapy session are a) using a coping card to put a problem-solving strategy into action, b) completing a worksheet for examining the evidence to modify automatic thoughts or schemas, and c) following a behavioral plan to increase pleasurable activities.
3. *Always follow up on homework assigned at a previous session.* When you review and discuss homework, you communicate that the task is important. But if you don't ask the patient about previously assigned homework, you may send a message that it is not useful enough to take up therapy time and therefore not worth the patient's effort. A common problem is getting caught up in discussion of new information and forgetting to review the homework from the previous session. To avoid this error, put homework review on each session's agenda.
4. *Be careful about using the term "homework."* Most adult patients will not have negative reactions to use of the word *homework*. They will understand that you are suggesting practical exercises that are likely to help them cope better with their problems. However, alternative terms for

homework may be useful when treating patients who are of school age or who have a negative view of their school experiences. If needed, you can call the assignment a self-help exercise. Or you can simply ask patients how they would like to use what they have learned in the session during their time between visits: "Now that you know how to recognize negative thoughts, how can you use this skill at home when upsetting things happen?" "How would you like to apply the activity schedule in your daily life?" "What kinds of opportunities do you see for using coping cards?"

Recovery

1. *Evaluate the acceptability and usefulness of the assignment.* Sometimes a task or exercise may seem like a good idea during the session but may become impractical or unnecessary after the patient has had time to think about it. If the patient says that she did not do the homework, ask if it is still worth doing. If the patient says that it is, revise the plan to make it more acceptable or useful. If the assignment is no longer necessary, drop it and move on to something else.

2. *Complete the missed homework during the session.* If the previously assigned homework is something that can be completed during a session, take time to work on it before developing any new assignments. Sometimes all that is necessary is for the therapist to help the patient get started on a task:

   > José wanted to apply for a job and needed to write a cover letter to accompany his résumé. He agreed to do this as homework, but when he got home he found that he had no idea how to start. During his next therapy session, José and his therapist brainstormed about what to say in the letter. With this information in hand, José was able to write the cover letter on his own before the next session.

3. *Evaluate negative thoughts about the homework task.* The negative thinking that comes with anxiety, depression, and other disorders can interfere with homework completion. For example, if the patient feels hopeless, he may be too discouraged to take action. If the homework is an exposure exercise, catastrophic thoughts can lead to avoidance of taking chances. Examples of maladaptive thoughts about homework include "I was never any good in school.... I can't do this"; "I have to do the homework perfectly or not at all"; "I can't do anything right...why should I try?" When you identify these types of reactions to homework assignments, you can work to modify the cognitions with thought records, examining the evidence, or other CBT

methods. Ask the patient to write down the conclusion of these exercises so that it can be reviewed if the negative thoughts return.

4. *Use homework noncompletion as a learning opportunity.* The reasons for noncompletion of homework can often provide good opportunities for CBT interventions. For example, the patient may report that problems with low energy, lack of confidence, procrastination, trouble organizing a daily schedule, or being overwhelmed with stressors may have interfered with doing homework. In each instance, the therapist can help the patient to identify and modify cognitive-behavioral pathology that undermines her ability to carry out the homework. There are dual benefits to using homework noncompletion as a target for therapy interventions: a) adherence with homework can be improved, and b) basic CBT skills can be practiced and enhanced.

Difficulty Eliciting Automatic Thoughts

Some patients may provide only cursory reports of events or may have difficulty verbalizing specific automatic thoughts. In these cases, therapists might feel compelled to help patients uncover the details of a story by completing sentences for them and making assumptions about what they are thinking or feeling. This strategy is usually a mistake. The clinician may not detect important cognitions, and patients may feel misunderstood if the therapist guesses incorrectly.

Prevention

1. *Let the patient tell a story about an upsetting event.* Listen for the automatic thoughts, paraphrase them to be certain you heard them correctly, and ask the patient to write the cognitions on a thought record. Unless the patient is a long-winded storyteller, allow him to fully explain events before asking him to identify specific automatic thoughts. If he has trouble verbalizing his automatic thoughts, ask him to visualize the event and describe what he sees.

2. *Explore the meanings of events.* When the patient does not know what is bothering him about a situation, ask what it was about the event that stirred up strong feelings. "What was it about her tone of voice that made you so angry? What was so irritating about that experience?" If the answer is "I don't know," give the patient time to think it over. Then try to help the patient understand the meaning of the event. The value of asking about the meanings of events is illustrated in the next example:

Trisha felt very angry when her father came into her garage and helped her with some shelves she was struggling to assemble. All he said to her was "Here, let me do it." Yet she found herself burning with rage. At first it made no sense to Trisha why an act of kindness would enrage her. However, when she thought about what his words meant to her, she was able to identify some intense negative thoughts about the situation. "He thinks I'm too stupid to do it myself. My parents have been doing things for me all my life, and I let them do it. They don't think I'm capable of figuring things out on my own. I want to be independent, but every time I try, they end up stepping in to help me. Maybe I am incompetent."

3. *Try to spot "hot" cognitions.* As noted in Chapter 5, "Working With Automatic Thoughts," intense emotions usually indicate that significant automatic thoughts have emerged. Therefore, efforts should be made to ask patients questions that stimulate emotion. Imagery can be used if the patient has difficulty recalling situations that were associated with automatic thoughts and significant emotional arousal.
4. *Ask about the person's actions during the upsetting event.* Work backward from behavior to cognitions by inquiring about what made a particular action seem reasonable or what alternatives might have been considered. For example, if the person took no action, ask, "If you could turn back time, what action do you wish you had taken? What was it about the event that kept you from doing that in the first place?"

Recovery

1. *Avoid asking forced-choice (i.e., yes/no, multiple-choice) questions.* When patients have difficulty producing automatic thoughts, it may be tempting to start asking forced-choice questions to draw out their reactions to situations. For example, you might ask: "Did it make you angry? Were you feeling down about it? Was it because you felt rejected?" If you find yourself asking these types of questions, rephrase them in an open-ended style: "What kinds of thoughts were stirred up by this event? How did you feel about yourself? What thoughts did you have about the other people in the situation?"
2. *Stay with a topic if it is important.* Don't give up prematurely if a patient has trouble identifying automatic thoughts. Sometimes a little extra effort or a different approach will allow you to uncover important streams of cognitions. Imagery or role play may help patients immerse themselves in scenes and recall salient automatic thoughts. Also, homework assignments to confront troublesome situations can bring out automatic thoughts that may not be apparent during therapy sessions.

3. *Record thoughts as close to a stressful event as possible.* Sometimes patients will say that they don't seem to have any thoughts that precede painful emotions; they just suddenly have a panic attack, some other form of anxiety, or a spell of sadness. Because it may be very difficult for these patients to remember any of their thoughts several days after the episode, it often helps to develop a homework assignment to identify immediately cognitions that are occurring during a panic attack or other emotional outpouring, and to either write them down or record them on audiotape. Then the automatic thoughts can be brought to the next therapy session for review and analysis.

4. *Use a checklist or other treatment adjuncts.* If other methods are not helpful in identifying automatic thoughts, consider using a checklist such as the Automatic Thoughts Questionnaire (Hollon and Kendall 1980) or the brief list provided in Chapter 5, "Working With Automatic Thoughts." You may also want to suggest self-help books or computerized methods of identifying automatic thoughts (Wright et al. 2004). Checklists, readings, and computerized CBT can provide valuable alternatives for recognizing automatic thoughts.

5. *Review the goal list.* After the patient has mastered the methods for controlling negative automatic thoughts and the presenting symptoms have improved, the patient may no longer be flooded with negative thoughts in response to stressful events. When you find that there are few or no negative thoughts to discuss in sessions, there is a good chance that the patient is making substantial progress. It may be time to work on other treatment goals. Review the patient's initial goal list and assess overall progress. Modify the goals as needed to reflect improvements. You may also want to consider discussing treatment completion and determining how many more sessions may be needed to achieve the goals of therapy.

Overly Verbal Patients

Some patients may want to use the majority of the session to tell detailed or rambling stories about stressful events instead of developing strategies to manage specific problems. This tendency may be especially common in individuals who have had previous experiences with nondirective therapy and have been encouraged to talk freely in an unstructured way. Other patients may have a natural inclination to be very talkative. Although free expression of thoughts and feelings is an overall strength for participating in therapy, there are occasions when the therapist will need to help the patient channel her conversations to fully benefit from the methods of CBT.

Prevention

1. *Socialize the patient to CBT.* During the first session, explain the collaborative nature of CBT. Ask the patient about prior therapy experiences and discuss how the problem-oriented approach of CBT might differ. Ask permission to interrupt the patient occasionally if an opportunity appears to sharpen the focus of therapy or teach a new skill.
2. *Address your own discomforts with interrupting patients.* Previous training in supportive, nondirective, or psychodynamically oriented therapy may make it difficult for some therapists to take an active role in interrupting patients and redirecting the flow of conversation. In addition, some therapists may have personality traits or background experiences that make them hesitant to interrupt others. If you find that you have difficulty asking patients to be more focused in their conversations, review this issue with a supervisor and practice polite ways to interrupt. For example, you might say, "Do you mind if I interrupt you? You just said something really important, and I want to know more about it." If the patient changes subjects before you have a chance to intervene, interrupt by saying, "Before you go on to tell me about your sister, I wonder if we could talk a little more about that last thing. You said something that really caught my attention, and I think I know how I might be able to help." Most patients will be cooperative and will allow you to speak, or will at least be curious about what you were going to suggest. If the patient jumps in and changes the subject again before you are through, stop her by saying, "I want to hear more about that, but I think it would be best if we finished up what we started before going on to a new topic."
3. *Teach the patient how to give brief summaries of events.* During the first few sessions of CBT, try to show patients how capsule summaries can be used to absorb the key points from a story they are telling or from a therapy intervention. Give brief summaries yourself to model ways of capturing the essence of a communication in a few sentences. Then ask the patient to do the same.

Recovery

1. *Balance session structure and open discussion.* When the patient routinely talks for the majority of the session about upsetting events, insufficient time may be left for interventions. Pause to explain again the interactive process of CBT and how you would like to teach the patient new skills for addressing recurring problems. If the patient is a natural storyteller and feels frustrated by the structured nature of CBT, budget a modest

amount of time for open discussions. In these cases, it is best if the majority of the effort is devoted to working on specific agenda items while some time is set aside for the patient to report on what has happened since the last visit. To enlist the patient's cooperation in such structuring of sessions, you might say something like the following: "You are wonderful at telling about your experiences. I appreciate learning about the people in your life and the problems you face. But I've found that I can get caught up in the details of the story and do not make enough time to teach you something new. The session ends before we have a chance to practice ways to deal with your problems. What I would like to suggest is that we both do a better job at setting aside enough time for the work of CBT. What do you think?"

2. *Rather than discourage a patient's ventilating, try to focus it.* Some patients will say that they just need to talk and do not wish to be interrupted or redirected. The patient may appreciate having someone to talk to about her life events or may have had positive therapy experiences in the past in which she was encouraged to ventilate feelings. One method to focus ventilating is to use the automatic thought record during the session. As the patient describes an event from her life, fill in the diary and share what you have written. Then teach the patient to use the thought recording technique to identify key automatic thoughts and emotions that are generated while ventilating.

Patients Who Are Stuck in a Behavior Pattern

Some behavior problems are difficult to change, particularly if they are habits that have been present for many years. In addition, symptoms of depression and anxiety can interfere with efforts to act differently. The following practical suggestions can help patients reverse problematic behavior patterns.

Prevention

1. *Discuss how the patient's current symptoms might interfere with his plans for changing behavior.* If the patient has depression, there is a good chance that low energy and motivation—hallmark symptoms of depression—could keep him from completing assignments. If anxiety is the problem, the individual may be too fearful to engage in exposure activities. If a limited attention span is the issue, he may not be able to complete lengthy reading assignments. Be mindful of how symptoms might interfere with treatment, and devise a strategy to work around them.

2. *Draw on the patient's strengths in designing interventions.* Identify interests, positive habits, supportive relationships, or other resources that can be used to change a long-standing behavior pattern. Could the patient's spiritual beliefs, attention to detail, or sense of humor help him see things differently and stick with a new plan? Many people find that doing things such as exercise or studying with a friend can be a way of overcoming procrastination.

3. *Look ahead for problems the patient may have in breaking old habits.* Anticipate factors that might interfere with the patient taking action. For example, if the patient watches television instead of tending to tasks, factor this into the action plan. Perhaps the behavior the patient wants to change should occur before the television is turned on in the morning. Or you might need to negotiate a behavioral contract to limit time spent in front of the television.

4. *Elicit and modify cognitions that are promoting procrastination, avoidance, or helplessness.* Some patients may have automatic thoughts or underlying schemas that are part of the problem. A young woman whom one of us treated was a chronic procrastinator. She had trouble completing assignments in school, following through with commitments, and sticking with plans. An important part of her therapy was working on a core belief that was driving her procrastination: "If I really try, I will fail. Then I will be exposed as the loser that I truly am."

5. *Encourage self-monitoring.* Good plans to overcome procrastination often include efforts to log the behaviors that the patient is trying to change. Data recording can reinforce positive movement, show the patient where he is having problems following the plan, and provide excellent material for discussion in therapy sessions. Examples of logs might include food diaries, records of physical exercise completed (e.g., time spent exercising, calories expended, type of exercise), or notes on efforts spent trying to find a new job.

6. *Use a graded approach.* As discussed in Chapter 6, "Behavioral Methods I: Improving Energy, Completing Tasks, and Solving Problems," difficult tasks can often be broken down into smaller steps. If the patient gains experience and confidence with less complex parts of the task, he may then be able to progress in a gradual fashion to achieve the overall behavioral goal.

Recovery

1. *Try again.* It is difficult to change old habits. Ask the patient if the behavior change that he planned is still a priority. If he says that it is, ask

him to try to implement the change again. Select a time and place for the action that has the greatest likelihood of success. Reach agreement that he will attempt the behavioral exercise more than once before the next therapy session.

2. *Use cognitive rehearsal.* Before the patient makes another attempt, ask him to imagine engaging in the new behavior and to describe, step by step, what he will do. Attend to potential obstacles along the way, and help prepare him for overcoming any roadblocks that could interfere with progress.

3. *Evaluate the advantages and disadvantages of changing the behavior pattern.* Create a grid with two columns, one labeled "Advantages" and the other "Disadvantages." Label one row with the behavior pattern under consideration (e.g., "Procrastination") and the other row indicating the alternative action (e.g., "Taking action"). Then ask the patient to identify the most important advantage and disadvantage of each option. Find a behavioral strategy that allows the patient to retain some advantages of the bad habit while gaining the main advantages of the good habit. Figure 9–1 provides an example of one patient's evaluation of the advantages and disadvantages of procrastination.

Progress Derailed by Environmental Stress

It is very common for patients with psychiatric illnesses to have significant psychosocial stressors in their lives such as family conflict, financial difficulties, school problems, legal issues, divorce, and serious medical conditions. Your efforts to achieve progress can be derailed when the focus of therapy must turn to crisis management and away from skills training. If there are many sources of stress in the patient's life, it is easy to get caught up in discussion of these topics and not find time to directly address the symptoms that brought the person to treatment.

Prevention

1. *Try not to get overwhelmed with the complexity of the patient's problems.* Monitor your own automatic thoughts about your ability to help the patient. Use the skills you are teaching the patient to control your own negative thinking. If you are discouraged by the complexity of the patient's life or are having hopeless thoughts, it will show in your demeanor and will affect your ability to help the patient solve her many problems.

	Advantages	Disadvantages
Procrastination	Less stress. I don't have to deal with it. It is easier. I don't have to fail. I can use my time for more enjoyable things.	I'm stressed out about the things I have to do. My house and office are a mess. I look like a loser to everyone. I don't fit in with people who have their act together. I hate myself for doing it.
Taking action	I can get things accomplished. I will feel better about myself. I can stop worrying about the things I used to avoid. My family would be proud of me.	There is too much to do. I will not be able to handle it. It will be stressful and unpleasant.

Figure 9–1. Patient evaluation of advantages and disadvantages of procrastination.

2. *Choose one target problem at a time.* Even if it means that other important problems or symptoms must be temporarily bypassed, it is usually best to stick with a targeted line of inquiry until you can start to see results. Try to keep focused on one problem rather than giving limited attention to various issues and not solving any. If the patient learns how to apply CBT methods in tackling one significant problem, she can then apply these skills when working on other issues and concerns.

3. *Teach problem-solving skills.* Problems such as neglecting to pay bills or failing to control unhealthy eating habits can accumulate or compound over time when a person is too ill or too overwhelmed to address them. Because the symptoms of depression and anxiety can include pessimism about the future and one's ability to cope with problems, patients can talk themselves out of taking control of their situation before they even try. A common complaint is "I don't know where to start." As discussed in Chapter 6, "Behavioral Methods I: Improving Energy, Completing Tasks, and Solving Problems," you can help patients take action by teaching them problem-solving methods such as prioritizing difficulties, setting effective goals, and organizing their daily schedule.

Recovery

1. *Regroup.* If you have become burdened or perplexed by the complexity of the patient's problems during a session, you can regroup by

summarizing out loud the challenges faced by the patient, helping the patient prioritize the problems on the list, and selecting a single focus for an intervention.

2. *Bring in reinforcements.* Therapists can become weighed down by the scope of some patients' psychosocial problems, particularly if the clinicians believe they have primary responsibility for solving the patients' difficulties. Find out who might be available in the patient's environment to assist with resolving psychosocial problems. When feeling overwhelmed with stress, patients can forget that other people might provide assistance if they knew of a need. Work through the patient's negative automatic thoughts about asking for help, and rehearse how to approach others for assistance.

3. *Use the past as a guide.* Find out what strategies the patient used in the past to cope with stress. There is a good chance that he has been through difficult times before and found a way out of them. If the person can recall past efforts at problem solving but lacks the self-confidence to take similar actions now, try to change the negative automatic thoughts by generating evidence for and evidence against his ability to use existing skills to cope with new problems.

Therapist Fatigue or Burnout

Psychotherapy is difficult work. It can be mentally taxing and emotionally stressful for all therapists regardless of experience. When you are new to the field and are not fully comfortable with the methods or confident in your skill, you can feel frustrated with patients who are not making progress. This can cause a temporary feeling of burnout and make you want to give up on patients, or give up on being a therapist altogether. If you can persevere through the training process until you have refined your skills and gained confidence, the temporary feeling of burnout is likely to dissipate. However, because of the mentally intensive nature of psychotherapy, therapists may periodically become fatigued with their work. There are several things you can do to prevent or limit the feeling of fatigue or burnout. A few examples are listed below.

Prevention

1. *Take care of your basic needs.* Busy therapists who are accustomed to working hard can drive themselves so relentlessly that they neglect their own personal daily needs. Telltale signs of this problem include running late in the morning so you don't take time for breakfast, over-

scheduling or being late between sessions so that there are no breaks between patients, and agreeing to see patients during a lunch hour. To be effective as a therapist, you must be mentally sharp, focused, and not distracted by competing physical and mental stressors. If you want to give your patients your best, schedule time to take care of yourself.

2. *Find your limits.* There is wide variety in the caseload that therapists can maintain and the number of hours of clinical practice they can conduct each day or each week without becoming overly fatigued. You have exceeded your limit when you find that you are too exhausted to be effective, too tired to do anything after work, disinterested in hearing about the problems of your family members or friends, or self-medicating after work to decompress from the day. Another indicator that you have exceeded your limit is when you no longer enjoy your work. Find your limits and create a daily schedule that allows you to function within these boundaries.

3. *Keep a healthy balance between your dedication to work and the rest of your life.* Develop a hobby or interest that adds variety to your schedule. Have other things to look forward to in your week in addition to your patients. Devote time to other things that are meaningful to you.

Recovery

1. *Rest.* Get enough sleep. Find relaxing activities that recharge your energy level. Schedule a long weekend or a vacation away from work to rest your mind and refuel your spirit. When you are not working, engage in activities that use a different set of cognitive skills or that are more physical in nature. This will give the empathic listening and problem-solving parts of your brain a short rest. Avoid thinking about work during this time off.

2. *Get supervision.* If you think your fatigue is focused on a specific patient, talk to a supervisor or colleagues about your work. If you are experiencing countertransference, discuss this issue in supervision and develop a strategy to manage the response. You may discover that you become more easily fatigued with a specific type of presenting problem. Perhaps you find certain illnesses or clusters of symptoms difficult or tedious to manage or do not yet possess the skills to treat them. For example, some clinicians do not like working with people who have substance abuse problems or personality disorders. If you find this kind of work unpleasant or uninteresting, consider limiting your practice to exclude such individuals. Find colleagues who specialize in these areas and refer patients to them.

3. *Learn something new.* Fatigue or burnout can be associated with doing the same thing with every patient. In CBT, there is a risk that methods for specific disorders can become so structured and similar to one another that you may find yourself becoming bored with the routine. If this is the case, learn something new. Take a class, read a book, or talk with other clinicians about their therapeutic approaches. As long as you stay within the conceptual model of CBT, there is an abundance of creative ways in which the methods can be applied. Examples might include a) implementing a new technique for a specific disorder (e.g., dialectical behavior therapy for borderline personality disorder, behavioral methods for eating disorders, or cognitive restructuring for psychoses; see Chapter 10, "Treating Chronic, Severe, or Complex Disorders"), b) using computer programs for CBT (see Chapter 4, "Structuring and Educating"), c) employing teaching devices such as marker boards or drawing materials, and d) suggesting self-help reading materials that encourage the patient to bring alternative ideas to treatment sessions.

Medication Regimen Nonadherence

Inconsistent use of medications is a common problem, particularly when pharmacotherapy regimens are lengthy or cause uncomfortable side effects. Therefore, if your patient's treatment plan includes taking psychotropic medications, it will be important for you to consider CBT methods that can improve adherence. Research on CBT and pharmacotherapy has demonstrated a significant positive effect in enhancing adherence with medication regimens (Cochran 1984; Kemp et al. 1996; Lecompte 1995).

When the clinician is a physician or nurse practitioner, CBT methods can be fully integrated with medication management skills to present a cohesive, comprehensive model for treatment. A significant emphasis of the therapy can be on understanding and adhering to the pharmacotherapy regimen. However, if you are not the treating physician, your role may be to help the patient communicate about medication regimen adherence with the prescriber.

Prevention

1. *Create a comfortable environment for discussing adherence.* Normalize adherence problems by letting the patient know that it is difficult for most people to stick with treatment for long periods of time. Do not pass judgment or be critical about inconsistencies in taking medica-

tion. To openly discuss her habits for taking medication, the patient has to feel comfortable reporting nonadherence. Thus, you will need to be an objective, nonthreatening listener.

2. *Anticipate obstacles to adherence.* Ask the patient if she has had any difficulty sticking with treatment in the past. Find out what has interfered with adherence. Some of the most common problems are a) forgetfulness or disorganization, b) feeling better, c) side effects, d) negative attitudes about medications, e) discouragement from others, and f) discomfort with the prescribing physician. Determine if any of these factors are currently present or could occur in the near future. When there are significant changes in a person's routine, schedule, or environment, inquire about how these changes might interfere with medication-taking behaviors.

3. *Create a plan for avoiding adherence problems.* Map out a written plan for overcoming each potential obstacle to adherence. Review the document periodically to determine if any modifications or additions are needed to maximize adherence. Shown in Figure 9–2 is an adherence plan that was developed for a person with bipolar disorder.

4. *Check for adherence frequently.* Don't assume that the patient is taking medications as prescribed, even when you believe you have an excellent therapeutic relationship. Monitor progress with adherence on a routine basis, not just when the patient is symptomatic. Ask open-ended questions that encourage the patient to give an honest report on her medication-taking behavior. There can be problems with questions such as "Are you taking all of your medication?" In an attempt to please you, the patient might say "Yes" when she is actually missing some doses. A better question to ask may be "How are you doing in taking your medication as planned?"

Recovery

1. *Assess the patient's automatic thoughts and core beliefs about taking medication.* If you detect maladaptive thoughts about medications (e.g., "People who take medications are weak"; "I'll get dependent on the drug"; "No one will trust me if they find out I'm taking this medication"; "I should be able to get better on my own"), you can use standard CBT methods such as psychoeducation, spotting cognitive errors, and examining the evidence to modify the cognitions. If you suspect that poor adherence is related to lack of acceptance of the diagnosis, make efforts to normalize and destigmatize the illness. You might also suggest readings that help explain the disorder.

Why I might not take medication	Solutions
I get up late, rush out of the house to go to work, and forget to take my medication.	Set the alarm clock every night. Place pills beside my toothbrush so that I remember to take them every day, even if I'm running late. (I always brush my teeth in the morning.)
I start to think that the medication brings me down and that I don't really need it.	Review the list I made with the doctor of the disadvantages of stopping medications. For example, I lose too much sleep and become irritable with everyone; I have lost control when manic and have gotten into financial trouble; I was fired from a job because I became manic.
I go on a trip and forget to take my medications with me.	Have a backup plan. Ask the doctor for samples, and store a few of them in my suitcase. Also, ask for an extra prescription I can keep in my wallet.
I begin to feel really good. I'm on a roll, and I forget to take the medication.	Agree to listen to my wife and my parents when they tell me I'm getting manic. Agree that it is OK for them to remind me to take medication. Keep medications in a weekly container so that my family will know if I'm taking the pills.

Figure 9–2. Sample medication adherence plan.

2. *Use simple behavioral strategies.* Work collaboratively with the patient to find behavioral plans that can reverse patterns of nonadherence. For example, pair medication taking with another routine activity that is done each day (e.g., suggest that pill taking become part of the patient's routine for preparing to go to bed each night), use reminder systems, or devise a behavioral contract.

3. *Help the patient talk about adherence with the prescribing clinician* (if that is not you). You can elicit automatic thoughts about taking medication and suggest that the patient write these down to tell the physician. Another strategy is to use role-play exercises to help the patient voice concerns about medication. In some situations, it may be helpful to ask the patient's permission to discuss adherence issues and plans with the medical practitioner.

4. *Set goals for improving adherence.* Identify the pattern of nonadherence. Does it occur with one but not all medications? Is it the morning dose that is usually forgotten? Focus on specific goals for improvement regarding the time of day or the type of medication that is taken less consistently.

Summary

Some of the more common problems encountered in delivering CBT include homework noncompletion, difficulty identifying automatic thoughts, overly verbal patients, being stuck in a negative behavior pattern, overwhelming environmental stress, therapist fatigue and burnout, and medication regimen nonadherence. We suggest that you carefully monitor your therapy efforts in managing these types of challenges and that you discuss your ideas for solutions with colleagues and supervisors. Each obstacle encountered in the delivery of CBT is an opportunity to learn more about therapy and enrich your clinical skills.

References

Cochran SD: Preventing medical noncompliance in the outpatient treatment of bipolar affective disorders. J Consult Clin Psychol 52:873–878, 1984

Hollon SD, Kendall PC: Cognitive self-statements in depression: development of an automatic thought questionnaire. Cognit Ther Res 4:383–395, 1980

Kemp R, Hayward P, Applewhaite G, et al: Compliance therapy in psychotic patients: randomised controlled trial. BMJ 312:345–349, 1996

Lecompte D: Drug compliance and cognitive-behavioral therapy in schizophrenia. Acta Psychiatr Belg 95:91–100, 1995

Wright JH, Wright AS, Beck AT: Good Days Ahead: The Multimedia Program for Cognitive Therapy. Louisville, KY, Mindstreet, 2004

10

Treating Chronic, Severe, or Complex Disorders

After completing your initial training in cognitive-behavior therapy (CBT)—which is usually best accomplished through supervised work with patients with major depressive disorder or one of the common anxiety disorders—it is time to gain experience working with patients with more complex problems. Since the 1980s, a number of research studies have documented the utility of CBT and related models of therapy for patients with severe, chronic, or treatment-resistant disorders such as bipolar disorder, borderline personality disorder, and schizophrenia.

For these populations of patients with conditions that are more difficult to treat, several common elements guide therapy. These include the following:

- The cognitive-behavioral model and all aspects of CBT are fully compatible with appropriate forms of pharmacotherapy.
- Regardless of the level of severity or impairment, the therapeutic relationship is characterized by the collaborative empirical stance.
- Therapy follows a coherent structure: each session begins with an agenda, and segments of sessions end with a brief summary and the opportunity for the patient to provide feedback before moving on to the next agenda item.
- Homework assignments build directly on the material addressed within sessions.

- Therapeutic strategies target aspects of problematic cognitions, affects, or behaviors.
- When indicated, family members and significant others may be invited to join the therapy team to facilitate progress in therapy.
- Outcomes are assessed and methods of therapy are adjusted to maximize the chances for improvement.

In this chapter, we briefly review CBT and related models of therapy that have been adapted for use with patients who have severe psychiatric conditions. The emphasis is on discussing empirical evidence for these approaches and providing general guidelines for working with patients with more complex or disabling illnesses. Books and treatment manuals for CBT of problems such as bipolar disorder, Axis II disorders, and schizophrenia are listed in Appendix 2, "Cognitive-Behavior Therapy Resources."

Severe, Chronic, and Treatment-Resistant Depressive Disorders

Traditional models for the treatment of depressive disorders either implicitly or explicitly suggest that severe or chronic depression is largely biological in nature and therefore is more likely to require somatic forms of therapy (American Psychiatric Association 1993; Rush and Weissenburger 1994; Thase and Friedman 1999). Although the results of some studies suggest that severely depressed outpatients may be less responsive to CBT than patients with milder depression (Elkin et al. 1989; Thase et al. 1991), severe depression is not a contraindication to CBT alone. In fact, a review of a large number of ambulatory studies found that more severely depressed patients respond as well to CBT as they do to pharmacotherapy with antidepressants (DeRubeis et al. 1999). In addition, a number of studies have demonstrated that the addition of CBT to pharmacotherapy resulted in significant improvement in the outcomes of patients with severe, recurrent, or chronic forms of major depressive disorder (Fava et al. 1998b; Keller et al. 2000; Thase et al. 1997).

Several modifications of standard CBT have been recommended for patients with markedly severe or chronic depressive disorders (Fava et al. 1998a; Thase and Howland 1994; Wright 2003), and comprehensive treatment protocols have been developed for hospitalized patients (Thase and Wright 1991; Wright et al. 1993). The modifications suggested by Fava et al. (1998a) and Wright (2003) are designed to adapt commonly used methods for CBT, as originally conceptualized by A.T.

Table 10–1. Potential targets for cognitive-behavior therapy of treatment-resistant depression

---

Hopelessness
Anhedonia
Low energy
Anxiety
Negative automatic thoughts
Maladaptive beliefs
Interpersonal problems
Nonadherence to pharmacotherapy

Beck and coworkers (1979) and described in this book, for treatment of chronic and severe depression. These modifications center on several observations: 1) patients with more-difficult-to-treat depression can become discouraged, hopeless, or burned out with treatment; 2) these individuals are usually plagued by slowed thinking and activity, low energy, and anhedonia; 3) symptoms such as anxiety and insomnia may require special attention; and 4) patients with treatment-resistant depression frequently have major interpersonal and social problems such as marital conflict, job loss, or financial difficulties. Targets for CBT are summarized in Table 10–1.

Fava and coworkers (1994, 1997, 1998a, 2002) conducted a series of studies that have shown good results of treatment modifications that include an early emphasis on behavioral strategies such as scheduling of activities and pleasant events to treat anhedonia and low energy, and exposure protocols for reducing anxiety. These researchers also use cognitive restructuring to address maladaptive thought patterns, and they also work intensively to help the patient carry out these interventions in therapy sessions and then in homework assignments. Wright (2003) suggested that addressing hopelessness and demoralization with CBT techniques and working with problem solving on social and interpersonal difficulties are additional potential targets for CBT of chronic or severe depression.

In treating these types of conditions, it is often useful to help patients identify fluctuations in mood during the course of a session, to demonstrate that change is possible and that coping strategies do have observable effects. To offset the tendency to discount stepwise gains as trivial, it is equally useful to suggest that small changes can have additive or cumulative effects. Relatively simple interventions such as thought stopping or other forms of therapeutic distraction may be used to help reduce the intensity of dysphoric ruminations. Suicidal ideation must be ad-

My Reasons for Living

- My children love me and would be hurt by my death.
- Others (parents and friends) also love me.
- When I am not depressed, there are things about life that I enjoy.
- When I am able to work at my "normal" capacity, I am a valued employee.
- My doctor says that I will respond to treatments and I may be better within a few weeks.

Figure 10–1.   Example: "Reasons for Living" coping card.

dressed early and vigorously; there may be no better means of rapidly helping a suicidal individual than to collaboratively develop a "Reasons for Living" list. An example of a list of reasons for living, reinforced by a coping card, is shown in Figure 10–1.

The timing and pacing of CBT sessions for severely depressed patients should fit their level of symptoms and capacity to participate in therapy. For some patients, twice-weekly sessions can be undertaken early in the treatment process. If concentration is a significant problem, frequent brief sessions of 20 minutes with a single intervention focus may be more helpful than conventional sessions of 45–50 minutes with two or three areas of intervention.

McCullough (1991, 2001) suggested a different set of modifications of CBT for work with patients with chronic depressive disorders. His approach, systematized as the Cognitive Behavioral Analysis System of Psychotherapy (CBASP; McCullough 2001), is based on observations that persons with chronic depression develop persistent difficulties with effectively defining and solving interpersonal problems. The CBASP method involves teaching patients how to effectively manage social situations, in addition to revising dysfunctional cognitions. However, less attention is paid to cognitive restructuring than in the approach recommended by Fava and colleagues (1994, 1997, 1998a, 2002). Readers interested in CBASP are referred to McCullough 2001 for a detailed explanation of how to implement this treatment approach for chronic depression.

Bipolar Disorder

Converging lines of evidence have established that 1) only a minority of patients with bipolar disorder respond to standard pharmacotherapies with long periods of remission; 2) nonadherence with medication regimens is a major cause of relapse; 3) stress increases the likelihood of illness episodes, whereas social support has beneficial effects; and 4) most people with bipolar disorder must cope with high levels of stress because of marital or relationship difficulties, unemployment or underemployment, periods of outright disability, and other problems that impair quality of life (Thase, in press). Thus there are multiple reasons to evaluate the potential benefits of CBT and other psychotherapies for people with bipolar disorder.

Comprehensive methods of CBT for bipolar disorder have been developed by Basco and Rush (1996) and Newman et al. (2002). CBT of bipolar disorder begins with the assumption that pharmacotherapy with a mood stabilizer (and possibly an atypical antipsychotic medication) is a necessary precondition for effective therapy; psychotherapy thus is viewed as having a treatment-enhancing or adjunctive role. Although an attempt might be made to use CBT alone for bipolar patients who refuse pharmacotherapy, we recommend concomitant use of lithium, divalproex, or another mood stabilizer with proven prophylactic effects.

Several studies have documented the efficacy of CBT when used in combination with standard medication regimens. In a small, very early trial, Cochran (1984) demonstrated that a brief course of CBT substantially improved treatment adherence. Subsequently, larger randomized trials were conducted by Scott and colleagues (2001) and Lam and colleagues (2003). In both trials, patients receiving CBT in addition to pharmacotherapy had fewer relapses and better functional outcomes than those who received pharmacotherapy alone.

The goals of CBT for bipolar disorder are summarized in Table 10–2. The first goal is to provide psychoeducation about bipolar disorder. The psychoeducational process includes teaching the patient about 1) the biology of bipolar disorder, 2) pharmacotherapy of this condition (if the clinician is a physician or nurse practitioner), 3) the effects of stress on symptom expression, and 4) the cognitive and behavioral elements of both depression and mania. Involvement in self-monitoring is the second goal of CBT for bipolar disorder. Early in the course of therapy, patients are taught to monitor several manifestations of their illness (e.g., symptoms, activities, and moods). Self-monitoring has several purposes: 1) to help separate features of the illness from normal moods and behaviors, 2) to evaluate how the illness affects the patient's day-to-day life, 3) to develop an early warning system for signs of relapse, and 4) and to identify targets for psychotherapeutic intervention. In addition, because people with bipolar disorder are prone to living rather chaotic, disorganized lifestyles, the simple act of monitoring daily activities can have a stabilizing effect.

Table 10–2.   Goals of cognitive-behavior therapy for bipolar disorder

---

1. Educate the patient and family about bipolar disorder.
2. Teach self-monitoring.
3. Develop relapse prevention strategies.
4. Enhance adherence to pharmacotherapy regimens.
5. Relieve symptoms with cognitive and behavioral methods.
6. Develop a plan for long-term management of bipolar disorder.

Developing relapse prevention strategies is a critical goal of CBT for bipolar disorder. One method used to promote relapse prevention is the production of a customized symptom summary worksheet that clearly delineates the changes that the patient and his family observe when he is beginning to exhibit early warning signs of mania or depression. This document is used as an early warning system to spot shifts in mood or behavior before a severe episode occurs. The therapist then helps the patient devise specific cognitive and behavioral strategies that are targeted toward limiting or reversing the progression of symptoms. For example, an inclination to think of schemes to rapidly make money might be countered with a list of advantages and disadvantages of pursuing these ideas and a behavioral plan to report these ideas to the therapist before taking any action.

A symptom summary worksheet for a man with hypomanic and manic symptoms is shown in Figure 10–2. This 33-year-old man with bipolar disorder was able to write down specific changes that typically occurred when he began to cycle into a manic episode. Detailed instructions on using this technique and other CBT methods for relapse prevention can be found in Basco and Rush (1996).

The fourth goal of CBT for bipolar disorder is one of the most important: enhancing adherence to pharmacotherapy regimens. From the CBT perspective, nonadherence is a common and understandable problem that almost inevitably complicates treatment of chronic disorders. Treatment adherence can be enhanced by identifying obstacles to regular medication taking and then systematically addressing these roadblocks (see Chapter 9, "Common Problems and Pitfalls: Learning From the Challenges of Therapy"). When the obstacle is the patient's negative thoughts and feelings about taking medication, standard CBT methods such as a thought change record or a pros-and-cons exercise can be used. Coping with unpleasant side effects can sometimes be enhanced by psychoeducation. However, changes in the medication regimen may also be required. Behavioral methods, including the use of reminder systems and pairing (taking medications at the same time and place as a routine activ-

Mild symptoms	Moderate symptoms	Severe symptoms
I start thinking of ideas and schemes to make a lot of money, but I don't do anything about it.	I am actively searching for inventions or investments that will make a lot of money or make me famous.	I try to withdraw funds from my IRA, get loans, or find some other way to get money to invest in a big deal or to start a new business.
I may have trouble falling asleep because my mind is full of ideas, but I try to sleep 7 hours so I can be rested to go to work.	I delay going to bed for 1–2 hours past the normal time. I'm too occupied with other things to want to sleep.	I only sleep 2–4 hours a night.
I feel more lively than usual. I don't care as much about my everyday problems. I want to party.	I go out a lot at night and ignore the work reports and planning documents I should be doing at home. I don't drink to excess, but I do have three to four beers when I go out with friends.	I spend way too much money entertaining, going out to fancy restaurants, etc. I've taken off on a whim to fly to New York City for a weekend and have charged beyond my limit on credit cards.
My mind feels more creative than usual. Ideas come easily.	My mind is going too fast. I don't pay attention to other people. I make mistakes at work because I don't pay attention.	I'm really juiced up. I'm thinking of so many different things that I'm jumping all over the place.
I'm a little more irritable than normal. I don't have much tolerance for people who I think are lazy. I'm more critical of my girlfriend than usual.	I get into lots of arguments at work and with my girlfriend.	I'm insufferable.
People I know well (my girlfriend and my mother) tell me that I need to slow down. They can tell that I'm speaking more rapidly or that I seem charged up.	I'm definitely speaking more rapidly and loudly than normal. Others seem to be irritated with the way that I talk to them.	I'm talking a mile a minute. I'm often impolite. I interrupt others and can shout in conversations.

Figure 10–2. A patient's symptom summary worksheet: an example of hypomanic and manic symptoms.

ity that is done each day—brushing teeth before going to bed, eating breakfast, getting dressed in the morning), are mainstays of the CBT approach to improving adherence.

The fifth goal is relief of symptoms through cognitive-behavioral interventions. The methods used for addressing depressive symptoms are the same as in standard CBT. In treating hypomanic symptoms, the therapist may focus on using behavioral strategies to treat insomnia, overstimulation, hyperactivity, and pressured speech. For example, CBT methods for insomnia (e.g., reducing distractions in the sleeping environment, providing education on healthy sleep patterns, and using thought stopping or diversions to decrease the rate of intrusive or racing thoughts) have been shown to be effective in restoring normal sleep patterns (Morin 2004). Efforts might also be made to set behavioral goals for cutting back on stimulating activities or monitoring and controlling the rate of speech.

Cognitive restructuring methods can be used to help hypomanic individuals identify and modify distorted thinking (e.g., Newman et al. 2002). Examples of these types of interventions are 1) spotting cognitive errors (e.g., magnifying one's sense of competence or power, ignoring risks, overgeneralizing from one positive feature to a more grandiose view of self), 2) using thought recording techniques to recognize expansive or irritating cognitions, and 3) listing advantages and disadvantages to evaluate the implications of holding on to an overly positive belief or prediction.

The sixth goal of CBT for bipolar disorder is to help patients with long-term illness management, including making lifestyle changes, facing and coping with stigma, and dealing more effectively with stressful life problems. In these capacities, CBT is distinguished from more supportive models of therapy by continued use of mood and activity monitoring, a stepwise approach to problem solving, and cognitive methods such as weighing the evidence to guide decision making.

Personality Disorders

Perhaps 30%–60% of patients with mood and anxiety disorders also meet criteria for one or more of the personality disorders listed in DSM-IV-TR (American Psychiatric Association 2000; Grant et al. 2005). Although not all studies are in agreement, Axis II conditions typically have negative prognostic implications and decrease the probability of response to treatment for mood and anxiety disorders, slow the temporal course of recovery, or increase the likelihood of relapse (Thase 1996). Interestingly, findings from several studies of CBT for major depressive disorder suggest that comorbid personality disorder may not adversely affect response to therapy (Shea et al. 1990; Stuart et al. 1992). Although these studies excluded patients with the most severe personality disorders, the findings do suggest that the structured methods used in CBT may be particularly well suited for patients with Axis II conditions.

The presence of a personality disorder is usually evident by the beginning of young adult life. However, personality pathology is not a static process and may be exaggerated by anxiety (e.g., increased avoidance), depression (e.g., increased dependence or exacerbation of borderline traits), or hypomania (e.g., increased narcissistic or histrionic traits). If your patient is presenting for treatment of an Axis I disorder, it is often useful to defer definitive assessment of Axis II conditions until after at least partial resolution of the mood or anxiety disorder. On occasion, compelling clinical evidence of a personality disorder is not apparent until after treatment has been initiated. In such cases, your treatment plan may need to be revised.

The CBT model for treatment of personality disorders focuses on the interactions between the individual's organizing beliefs or schemas that guide behavior, dysfunctional (and typically excessive) interpersonal strategies, and environmental influences (A.T. Beck and Freeman 1990; J.S. Beck 1997). Personality disorders are viewed as having their origins in adverse developmental experiences. Young (1990) outlined five thematic areas: 1) disconnection and rejection, 2) impaired autonomy and performance, 3) impaired limits, 4) other-directedness, and 5) overvigilance and inhibition.

Therapy of personality disorders generally uses many of the same methods developed for treatment of mood and anxiety disorders, but with a greater emphasis on schema work and on developing more effective coping strategies (J.S. Beck 1997). Other differences between CBT for treatment of personality disorders and CBT for treatment of depression and anxiety are the following: 1) the duration of therapy is usually much longer (i.e., a year or more); 2) more attention is paid to the therapeutic relationship and to transference reactions in working toward change; and 3) repeated practice of CBT methods is needed to modify chronic problems with self-concept, relationships with others, and emotional regulation and social skills.

Outlined in Table 10–3 are some of the predominant core beliefs, compensatory beliefs, and associated behavioral strategies common to specific personality disorders. Once a problematic schema or core belief is identified, CBT strategies such as examining the evidence and considering alternative explanations can be implemented.

Linehan's (1993) dialectical behavior therapy (DBT) is one of the principal adaptations of CBT for personality disorders. Developed specifically for treatment of individuals with borderline personality disorder,

Table 10–3. Personality disorders: beliefs and strategies

Personality disorder	Core belief about self	Belief about others	Assumptions	Behavioral strategy
Avoidant	I'm undesirable.	Other people will reject me.	If people know the real me, they'll reject me. If I put on a façade, they may accept me.	Avoid intimacy
Dependent	I'm helpless.	Other people should take care of me.	If I rely on myself, I'll fail. If I depend on others, I'll survive.	Rely on other people
Obsessive-compulsive	My world can go out of control.	Other people can be irresponsible.	If I'm not totally responsible, my world could fall apart. If I impose rigid rules and structure, things will turn out OK.	Control others rigidly
Paranoid	I'm vulnerable.	Other people are malicious.	If I trust other people, they will harm me. If I am on my guard, I can protect myself.	Be overly suspicious
Antisocial	I'm vulnerable.	Other people are potentially exploitive.	If I don't act first, I can be hurt. If I can exploit first, I can be on top.	Exploit others

Table 10–3. Personality disorders: beliefs and strategies *(continued)*

Personality disorder	Core belief about self	Belief about others	Assumptions	Behavioral strategy
Narcissistic	I'm inferior. (The manifest compensatory belief is "I'm superior.")	Other people are superior. (The manifest compensatory belief is "Others are inferior.")	If others regard me in a nonspecial way, it means they consider me inferior. If I achieve my entitlements, it shows I'm special.	Demand special treatment
Histrionic	I'm nothing.	Other people may not value me for myself alone.	If I am not entertaining, others won't be attracted to me. If I am dramatic, I'll get others' attention and approval.	Entertain
Schizoid	I'm a social misfit.	Other people have nothing to offer me.	If I keep my distance from others, I'll make out better. If I try to have relationships, they won't work out.	Distance self from others
Schizotypal	I am defective.	Other people are threatening.	If I sense that others are feeling negatively toward me, it must be true. If I'm wary of others, I can divine their true intentions.	Assume hidden motives

Table 10–3. Personality disorders: beliefs and strategies (*continued*)

Personality disorder	Core belief about self	Belief about others	Assumptions	Behavioral strategy
Borderline personality disorder	I'm defective. I'm helpless. I'm vulnerable. I'm bad.	Other people will abandon me. People can't be trusted.	If I depend on myself, I won't survive. If I trust others, they'll abandon me. If I depend on others, I'll survive but ultimately be abandoned.	Vacillate in extremes of behavior

Source.   Adapted with permission from Beck JS: "Cognitive Approaches to Personality Disorders," in *American Psychiatric Press Review of Psychiatry*, Vol. 16. Edited by Dickstein LJ, Riba MB, Oldham JM. Washington, DC, American Psychiatric Press, 1997, pp. 73–106. Copyright 1997 American Psychiatric Press. Used with permission.

DBT is distinguished by four key features: 1) acceptance and validation of one's behavior in the moment, 2) emphasis on identifying and treating therapy-interfering behaviors, 3) use of the therapeutic relationship as an essential vehicle for behavior change, and 4) a focus on dialectical processes (defined below in this section). Evidence from randomized, controlled clinical trials (Bohus et al. 2004; Linehan et al. 1991; Robins and Chapman 2004) that DBT can effectively reduce self-injurious and parasuicidal behavior has encouraged an expanding use of these methods in clinical practice. More recently, DBT has been successfully adapted for work with patients with substance abuse and eating disorders in addition to Axis II pathology (Linehan et al. 2002; Palmer et al. 2003).

The term *dialectical* helps to define and name DBT. Linehan (1993) chose this term to describe a holistic approach to psychopathology, drawing heavily on both Western and Eastern philosophies. Rather than viewing dysfunctional behavior as simply a symptom of an illness, the DBT approach follows the principle that even very problematic behavior serves certain functions. For example, splitting between various helpers or care providers may minimize (at least in the short run) the chances for receiving unwelcome, critical feedback and may maximize the chances of obtaining a desired outcome. A similar strategy is sometimes referred to in the business world as "playing both ends against the middle." Progress in therapy involves helping patients to recognize their ultimate goals and to be able to consider, and eventually implement, alternative, more socially acceptable methods to accomplish these goals.

DBT is also directed at coaching the patient on ways of gaining a better sense of balance between competing goals; for example, between acceptance and change, flexibility and stability, or eliciting nurturance and obtaining autonomy. Strategies pertaining to mindfulness are emphasized to help achieve these goals. The concept of *mindfulness* refers to teaching patients to better focus on the activity of the moment (i.e., to observe, describe, and participate), rather than being overwhelmed by strong emotions (Linehan 1993). Therapists also use behavioral methods such as relaxation training, thought stopping, and breathing retraining to assist patients with managing painful affects and regulating their emotional responses. In addition, social skills training strategies, including cognitive and behavioral rehearsal, are employed to help patients learn more effective methods to cope with interpersonal disputes.

Substance Use Disorders

Evidence regarding the utility of cognitive and behavioral therapies for substance use disorders (SUDs) has slowly emerged since the mid-1980s (see, e.g., Woody and Munoz 2000). Although there have been relatively few trials utilizing the fully developed CBT model of A.T. Beck and co-workers (1993), a number of studies document the utility of behavioral methods such as contingency management (Higgins et al. 1991, 1994), social skills training (Monti et al. 1993; Project MATCH Research Group 1998), and relapse prevention (Carroll et al. 1994). Beck's model of treatment was found to have a significant effect among methadone-maintained heroin addicts with higher levels of psychopathology (although not among those with lower levels of psychiatric symptoms; see Woody et al. 1984). However, little added benefit was documented in the National Institute on Drug Abuse Collaborative Cocaine Treatment Study, in which individual sessions of CBT were added to group chemical dependence counseling (Crits-Christoph et al. 1999). In fact, both CBT and a second form of professional psychotherapy (psychodynamically focused supportive and expressive therapy) were significantly less effective than individual drug counseling, even among the subset of patients with higher levels of psychiatric symptoms (Crits-Christoph et al. 1999). In retrospect, it is likely that the cognitive and psychodynamic therapists who participated in this study lacked sufficient experience working with this multiply disadvantaged, inner-city patient population.

With these caveats in mind, the interested reader will find more detailed descriptions of CBT for SUDs in publications by A.T. Beck and co-workers (1993) and Thase (1997). Illustrated in Figure 10–3 is the highly interdependent and reciprocal nature of the affects, behaviors, and cognitions associated with substance use. Although there are important sociodemographic, physiological, and clinical differences among the various SUDs, the cognitive-behavioral model posits that a common underlying process links the act of using intoxicating substances with underlying beliefs, cue-elicited urges and cravings, and negative automatic thoughts (A.T. Beck et al. 1993).

Several important tasks precede the initiation of formal therapy with CBT for substance abuse. First, if the SUD is characterized by a potentially dangerous withdrawal syndrome, enrollment in a medically supervised detoxification program may be necessary. Second, the patient's readiness for change should be assessed (Prochaska and DiClemente 1992). Motivation for therapy should be understood as occurring on a continuum, ranging from precontemplation (i.e., "I don't have a problem—I simply got caught driving after drinking a little too much") to contemplation to preparation to action. The methods of motivational interviewing (Miller et al. 2004; Strang and McCambridge 2004) are particularly well suited to help patients move from the precontemplation and contemplation stages to the preparation and action stages. A third

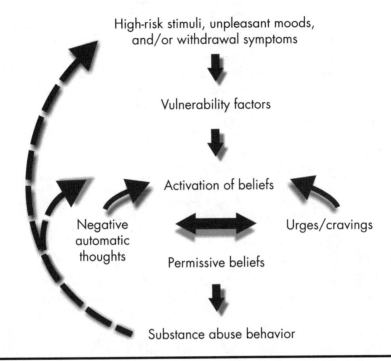

Figure 10–3. Cognitive-behavioral model of substance abuse.

Source. Adapted with permission from Thase ME: "Cognitive-Behavioral Therapy for Substance Abuse," in *American Psychiatric Press Review of Psychiatry*, Vol. 16. Edited by Dickstein LJ, Riba MB, Oldham JM. Washington, DC, American Psychiatric Press, 1997, pp. 45–71. Copyright 1997 American Psychiatric Press. Used with permission.

precondition is to establish a sobriety contract. Specifically, patients should commit to not coming to sessions under the influence of drugs or alcohol, and therapists need to learn to be comfortable saying "no—not today" when this contract is violated.

An important aspect of the CBT model is to help the patient recognize that urges and cravings to drink alcohol or use drugs are often associated with activation of relevant beliefs about drug or alcohol abuse. Cognitions related to substance abuse can occur almost instantaneously in response to personally relevant cues (i.e., the "persons, places and things" made popular by Alcoholics Anonymous). Although the distinction is somewhat artificial, urges can be conceptualized as the cognitive and behavioral predispositions to use drugs or alcohol, whereas cravings are the affective and physiological experiences that accompany the urges. In addition to situational cues, such as driving past a bar or seeing a television advertisement, urges and cravings can also be triggered by daydreams,

Table 10–4.   Beliefs about substance abuse

I don't have any control over craving.
Once it starts, the only way to cope with craving is to use.
I've passed the point of no return—I'll never be able to stop drinking.
You need willpower not to drink, and I don't have it.
I can't have fun without getting high.
It doesn't matter if I stop using—no one cares.
I can't cope without drinking.
My life is already ruined—I might as well get high.
No one can push me around—I'll quit when I'm ready.

Source.   Reprinted with permission from Thase ME: "Cognitive-Behavioral Therapy for Substance Abuse," in *American Psychiatric Press Review of Psychiatry*, Vol. 16. Edited by Dickstein LJ, Riba MB, Oldham JM. Washington, DC, American Psychiatric Press, 1997, pp. 45–71. Copyright 1997 American Psychiatric Press. Used with permission.

memories, or dysphoric emotions (most commonly anger, anxiety, sadness, or even boredom). Examples of beliefs relevant to the onset and maintenance of SUDs are provided in Table 10–4.

As the frequency and intensity of substance abuse increases, further cognitive changes can play a role in the evolution of the disorder. For example, there may be a tendency to devalue beliefs about more conventional mainstream goals and pursuits, including the desirability of maintaining the love, support, and approval of significant others. Similarly, beliefs about the adverse consequences of drugs and alcohol tend to be minimized, and attitudes pertaining to the positive effects of drinking or drug use are exaggerated. Secondary or *permissive* beliefs (e.g., "I can get high this one last time and can restart working on my sobriety program tomorrow" and "Once I start using, I can't stop—so I might as well go ahead and enjoy the high") also tend to be developed. Such beliefs help to explain the all-too-common tendency for a single use or lapse to spiral into a full-blown relapse.

Therapy thus proceeds down two simultaneous tracks: 1) achieving and maintaining sobriety, and 2) identifying and modifying the relevant beliefs that predispose to and maintain problematic substance use (see A.T. Beck et al. 1993). As success is gained in these areas, additional longer-range therapy goals may be addressed, including lifestyle and vocational changes. The cornerstone of successful CBT for substance abuse is relapse prevention (Marlatt and Gordon 1985). Relapse prevention strategies include both behavioral strategies to minimize the likelihood of encountering urges and cravings, and cognitive restructuring exercises to counter distorted negative thoughts about drinking or drug use. It is also usually a good idea to encourage patients to participate in self-help programs such as Alcoholics Anonymous.

Eating Disorders

CBT has become accepted as one of the primary methods of treatment for eating disorders (American Psychiatric Association Work Group on Eating Disorders 2000; Fairburn 1981; Garner and Bemis 1985; Mitchell and Peterson 1997). Strong evidence of efficacy has emerged from controlled studies of bulimia nervosa (Agras et al. 2000; Wilson 1999) and binge eating disorder (Agras et al. 1994; Ricca et al. 2000). In several studies, CBT was found to have additive effects when used in combination with antidepressant medications (Agras et al. 1992; Mitchell et al. 1990; Walsh et al. 1997). However, the effectiveness of CBT for anorexia nervosa has not yet been established (see, e.g., American Psychiatric Association 2000).

The CBT model for treating eating disorders is based on the notion that dysfunctional beliefs about slimness, and resulting dissatisfaction with body shape and weight, drive and maintain abnormal eating behavior and associated features such as purging and abuse of laxatives, diuretics, and diet pills. Contemporary societal standards that reinforce unrealistic goals regarding slimness have interacted with individual vulnerabilities (e.g., perfectionism, difficulty regulating affects, or propensity for depression) to cause a substantial increase in the incidence of these conditions.

Before working with an individual with an eating disorder, you may find it helpful to review the results of the classic study by Keys and colleagues (Keys 1950; Taylor and Keys 1950), which examined the effects of semistarvation on the attitudes and behaviors of healthy young men. Although these volunteers had virtually no risk of spontaneously developing an eating disorder, during the course of marked caloric restriction and significant weight loss, they developed preoccupations with food, diminished libido, mood and sleep disturbances, and cold intolerance. When the experimental caloric restriction ended, binge-eating behavior, food hoarding, and disturbed hunger and satiety cues developed. Most of the subjects regained more weight than they had lost, and it took weeks for them to fully restabilize. These observations underscore the fact that whatever the individual's vulnerability, the process of starvation and disordered eating behavior can play a significant role in maintaining an eating disorder.

The CBT approach is necessarily multimodal and includes nutritional counseling in addition to psychoeducation, self-monitoring, and cognitive and behavioral interventions. It is generally a good idea to work with an experienced dietician. An initial goal of treatment is to collaboratively determine a target weight range and meal plan. Although the relatively high normative values of the Metropolitan Life Insurance Company (1983) weight charts often elicit the equivalent of "sticker shock," it is imperative that a realistic goal be identified and a consistent method for monitoring weight be implemented. It is usually sufficient to obtain a weekly weight measurement. A meal plan generally consists of three regular meals and at least two snacks, with calories divided to minimize hunger cues. In the course of negotiating these terms of treatment, you will have ample opportunity to discuss any of the patient's concerns that the plan will backfire. Moreover, sharing the facts about the futility of common strategies presumed to facilitate weight loss, such as purging or using laxatives, is an important aspect of psychoeducation.

Self-monitoring initially entails keeping track of mealtimes and problem eating behavior, as well as potential environmental cues and triggers. Subsequently, three-column worksheets are used to help establish the links between negative thoughts, dysphoric affects, and problem eating behavior. Various strategies are used to either change or, if necessary, avoid responses to cues. Response prevention (see Chapter 7, "Behavioral Methods II: Reducing Anxiety and Breaking Patterns of Avoidance") is an important tool to help patients learn to prolong the interval between the urge (i.e., to binge, purge, or restrict) and the problematic behavior. Cognitive restructuring exercises are then employed to help patients cope with distorted negative thoughts about the consequences of not engaging in disordered eating behavior.

Schizophrenia

Schizophrenia is associated with a significantly greater likelihood of disability and a lower probability of the occurrence of periods of sustained and complete remission than most other severe psychiatric disorders, including bipolar I disorder (American Psychiatric Association 1997). The chronic nature of this devastating illness has provided impetus for the development of adjunctive psychosocial therapies. This need has persisted despite the introduction of a newer generation of antipsychotic drugs.

There is a relatively long history of research evaluating behavioral approaches to schizophrenia, including both contingency management strategies (Paul and Lentz 1977) and social skills training (Kazdin 1977; Liberman et al. 1998). Although they initially lagged behind, a number of applications of Beck's model of therapy had emerged by the mid-

1990s (Garety et al. 1994; Kingdon and Turkington 2004; Perris 1989; Scott and Wright 1997). There is now strong evidence from a series of clinical trials that individual CBT has significant effects in reducing both positive and negative symptoms of schizophrenia (A. T. Beck and Rector 2000; Sensky et al. 2000; Turkington et al. 2004).

Just as when using CBT in bipolar affective disorder, therapy should not be initiated until the patient has begun to stabilize on psychotropic medication. Sessions may be brief at the beginning. In some cases, two or three 20-minute sessions for a week or two may be more helpful than a single 45- or 50-minute session. It is also reasonable to anticipate that an optimal course of therapy will be longer than would be indicated for major depressive disorder or panic disorder.

Beyond establishing a therapeutic relationship, initial goals usually include psychoeducation about the disorder (including eliciting the patient's beliefs about the nature of schizophrenia and its treatment), increased involvement in activities, and improved adherence to pharmacotherapy regimens. As therapy progresses, attention shifts to identifying and modifying delusions and helping patients reduce or cope with hallucinations. Delusions can be viewed as an extreme form of the logical error of *jumping to conclusions*, in that the individual draws inferences on the basis of an incomplete assessment of facts and ignores or minimizes disconfirming evidence. If a collaborative therapeutic relationship can be established, the patient may be able to benefit from using logical analysis methods such as examining the evidence and searching for alternative solutions.

Presented in Figure 10–4 is an example of an exercise in examining the evidence completed by a 27-year-old man with schizophrenia. Ted had been doing volunteer work in the office of a community care center and had developed delusions about this environment. One of the triggers for these delusions was the appearance of a daily message on his computer screen. Although the daily message—typically a humorous quotation— was sent to every computer in the facility, Ted interpreted the messages in a delusional way. He had also begun to think that there was a plot by the Mafia or a foreign intelligence agency to take over the community care center. The technique of examining the evidence helped him recognize the distortions in his thinking and develop an alternative way of seeing the situation. In this case, Ted was encouraged to label the delusion as a *troubling thought* and to then apply standard CBT methods to test this cognition.

In treating hallucinations, it is usually helpful to introduce a *normalizing rationale*, namely, that nearly everyone will experience hallucinations under extreme circumstances (e.g., drug intoxication or marked sleep deprivation; Kingdon and Turkington 2004). This concept can help persons

Troubling thought: The Mafia or a foreign intelligence agency has infiltrated this office and is controlling everything.

Evidence for this thought:	Evidence against this troubling thought:
1. Computer messages are suspicious.	1. Computer messages are sent to everyone's computer. They are just witty sayings or jokes. They probably don't mean anything.
2. Two employees were fired last week	2. The people who got fired were always missing work.
3. There seem to be listening devices implanted in the TV monitors.	3. I took apart a TV and couldn't find anything suspicious. I tend to get paranoid.
4. I don't have any close friends at the center. People rarely talk to me.	4. It is true that I don't have many friends, but that doesn't mean that there is a plot to take over the center. I like doing this job, and everyone has treated me well.

Alternative thoughts: I know that I have a chemical imbalance that makes me get paranoid. Sitting in front of a computer for a couple hours a day has made me more suspicious. This job is worth my trying to calm my fears.

Figure 10–4. Examining the evidence for delusions: Ted's example.

with schizophrenia feel less stigmatized and be willing to look at possible environmental influences that could be aggravating hallucinations or to explore alternative explanations for hallucinations (to replace concepts such as "It's the devil"; "God is talking to me"; or "A woman's voice is torturing me"). The general goals in treating hallucinations with CBT are to help patients 1) accept a rational explanatory model for hallucinations (e.g., the normalizing rationale or a biological vulnerability), and 2) develop methods of reducing or limiting the impact of hallucinations.

One of the most helpful strategies for working with hallucinations is to generate a list of behaviors that either quiet the voices or make them less intrusive or commanding. The patient might also benefit from making a list of activities that worsen the voices. She can then develop a behavioral plan to increase helpful behaviors and decrease activities that amplify the hallucinations. An example of such a list of behaviors is presented in Figure 10–5. Barbara, a 38-year-old woman with schizophrenia, made this list of behaviors that helped her manage voices. She was able to identify a number of useful strategies, including diversionary activities, coaching herself on the nature of her illness (e.g., "I have a chemical imbalance, and I don't need to pay attention to the voices"), and an imagery technique that she designed herself without prompting from her therapist. Her plan also included efforts to learn how to better manage the situations and issues that appeared to aggravate her hallucinations.

Actions that make the voices softer or make them go away:	Actions that stimulate the voices or make them louder:
1. Listening to soothing music 2. Doing craft projects 3. Imagining that the voices are going into a closet in my house, a blanket is placed over the voices, and the door is locked 4. Doing volunteer work at my church 5. Reading a magazine or a book 6. Telling myself I have a chemical imbalance and I don't need to pay attention to the voices 7. Going to group therapy at the day treatment center	1. Arguments with my boyfriend or family members 2. Sleeping poorly 3. Forgetting to take medication 4. Watching violent or disturbing movies or TV shows

Figure 10–5. Actions that make voices better or worse: Barbara's example.

Negative symptoms can be approached with activity scheduling, graded task assignments, behavioral rehearsal, skills training, and related strategies. However, experts in the treatment of schizophrenia with CBT often recommend a "go-slow" approach in which the patient is given plenty of time to begin making changes in symptoms such as social isolation, withdrawal, and lack of initiative (Kingdon and Turkington 2004). You should keep in mind that even though negative symptoms may well reflect underlying neuropathology, individuals who have experienced even more debilitating forms of brain injury, including stroke or multiple sclerosis, can learn to use compensatory coping strategies in systematic approaches to rehabilitation.

Summary

Cognitive-behavioral methods have been developed and tested for a broad range of severe psychiatric disorders such as treatment-resistant depression, bipolar disorder, personality disorders, and schizophrenia. In addition, CBT techniques are a first-line treatment for bulimia nervosa and can provide useful tools for management of substance abuse problems. Although many of the standard cognitive and behavioral methods for depression and anxiety can also be used in the treatment of conditions that are more difficult to treat, specific modifications are recommended for advanced applications of CBT. In this chapter, we described empirical research that supports the use of CBT for chronic and severe mental illnesses, and we briefly detailed some of the strategies that can be used to meet the challenges of working with these conditions. In Chapter 11, "Building Competence in Cognitive-Behavior Therapy," we outline additional readings, workshops, and clinical supervision that can be used to build expertise in using CBT for severe psychiatric disorders.

References

Agras WS, Rossiter EM, Arnow B, et al: Pharmacologic and cognitive-behavioral treatment for bulimia nervosa: a controlled comparison. Am J Psychiatry 149:82–87, 1992

Agras WS, Telch CF, Arnow B: Weight loss, cognitive-behavioral, and desipramine treatments in binge eating disorder: an additive design. Behav Ther 25:225–238, 1994

Agras WS, Walsh T, Fairburn CG, et al: A multicenter comparison of cognitive-behavioral and interpersonal psychotherapy for bulimia nervosa. Arch Gen Psychiatry 57:459–466, 2000

American Psychiatric Association: Practice guideline for major depressive disorder in adults. Am J Psychiatry 150 (suppl):1–26, 1993

American Psychiatric Association: Practice guideline for the treatment of patients with schizophrenia. Am J Psychiatry 154 (suppl):1–63, 1997

American Psychiatric Association: Diagnostic and Statistical Manual of Mental Disorders, 4th Edition, Text Revision. Washington, DC, American Psychiatric Association, 2000

American Psychiatric Association Work Group on Eating Disorders: Practice guideline for the treatment of patients with eating disorders (revision). Am J Psychiatry 157 (1 suppl):1–39, 2000

Basco MR, Rush AJ: Cognitive-Behavioral Therapy for Bipolar Disorder. New York, Guilford, 1996

Beck AT, Freeman A: Cognitive Therapy of Personality Disorders. New York, Guilford, 1990

Beck AT, Rector NA: Cognitive therapy for schizophrenia: a new therapy for a new millennium. Am J Psychother 54:291–300, 2000

Beck AT, Rush AJ, Shaw BF, et al: Cognitive Therapy of Depression. New York, Guilford, 1979

Beck AT, Wright FD, Newman CF, et al: Cognitive Therapy of Substance Abuse. New York, Guilford, 1993

Beck JS: Cognitive approaches to personality disorders, in American Psychiatric Press Review of Psychiatry, Vol 16. Edited by Dickstein LJ, Riba MB, Oldham JM. Washington, DC, American Psychiatric Press, 1997, pp 73–106

Bohus M, Haaf B, Simms T, et al: Effectiveness of inpatient dialectical behavioral therapy for borderline personality disorder: a controlled trial. Behav Res Ther 42:487–499, 2004

Carroll KM, Rounsaville BJ, Gordon LT, et al: Psychotherapy and pharmacotherapy for ambulatory cocaine abusers. Arch Gen Psychiatry 51:177–187, 1994

Cochran SD: Preventing medical noncompliance in the outpatient treatment of bipolar affective disorders. J Consult Clin Psychol 52:873–878, 1984

Crits-Christoph P, Siqueland L, Blaine J, et al: Psychosocial treatments for cocaine dependence: results of the National Institute on Drug Abuse Collaborative Cocaine Treatment Study. Arch Gen Psychiatry 56:493–502, 1999

DeRubeis RJ, Gelfand LA, Tang TZ, et al: Medication versus cognitive behavior therapy for severely depressed outpatients: mega-analysis of four randomized comparisons. Am J Psychiatry 156:1007–1013, 1999

Elkin I, Shea MT, Watkins JT, et al: National Institute of Mental Health Treatment of Depression Collaborative Research Program: general effectiveness of treatments. Arch Gen Psychiatry 46:971–982, 1989

Fairburn C: A cognitive behavioural approach to the treatment of bulimia. Psychol Med 11:707–711, 1981

Fava GA, Grandi S, Zielezny M, et al: Cognitive behavioral treatment of residual symptoms in primary major depressive disorder. Am J Psychiatry 151:1295–1299, 1994

Fava GA, Savron G, Grandi S, et al: Cognitive-behavioral management of drug-resistant major depressive disorder. J Clin Psychiatry 58:278–282, 1997

Fava GA, Rafanelli C, Cazzaro M, et al: Well-being therapy: a novel psychotherapeutic approach for residual symptoms of affective disorders. Psychol Med 28:475–480, 1998a

Fava GA, Rafanelli C, Grandi S, et al: Prevention of recurrent depression with cognitive behavioral therapy: preliminary findings. Arch Gen Psychiatry 55:816–820, 1998b

Fava GA, Ruini C, Rafanelli C, et al: Cognitive behavior approach to loss of clinical effect during long-term antidepressant treatment: a pilot study. Am J Psychiatry 159:2094–2095, 2002

Garety PA, Kuipers L, Fowler D, et al: Cognitive behavioural therapy for drug-resistant psychosis. Br J Med Psychol 67 (pt 3):259–271, 1994

Garner DM, Bemis KM: Cognitive therapy for anorexia nervosa, in Handbook of Psychotherapy for Anorexia Nervosa and Bulimia. Edited by Garner DM, Garfinkel PE. New York, Guilford, 1985, pp 513–572

Grant BF, Hasin DS, Stinson FS, et al: Co-occurrence of 12-month mood and anxiety disorders and personality disorders in the US: results from the national epidemiologic survey on alcohol and related conditions. J Psychiatr Res 39:1–9, 2005

Higgins ST, Delaney DD, Budney AJ, et al: A behavioral approach to achieving initial cocaine abstinence. Am J Psychiatry 148:1218–1224, 1991

Higgins ST, Budney AJ, Bickel WK: Applying behavioral concepts and principles to the treatment of cocaine dependence. Drug Alcohol Depend 34:87–97, 1994

Kazdin AE: The Token Economy: A Review and Evaluation. New York, Plenum, 1977

Keller MB, McCullough JP, Klein DN, et al: A comparison of nefazodone, the cognitive behavioral-analysis system of psychotherapy, and their combination for the treatment of chronic depression. N Engl J Med 342:1462–1470, 2000

Keys A: The residues of malnutrition and starvation. Science 112:371–373, 1950

Kingdon DG, Turkington D: Cognitive Therapy of Schizophrenia. New York, Guilford, 2004

Lam DH, Watkins ER, Hayward P, et al: A randomized controlled study of cognitive therapy for relapse prevention for bipolar affective disorder: outcome of the first year. Arch Gen Psychiatry 60:145–152, 2003

Liberman RP, Wallace CJ, Blackwell G, et al: Skills training versus psychosocial occupational therapy for persons with persistent schizophrenia. Am J Psychiatry 155:1087–1091, 1998

Linehan MM: Cognitive-Behavioral Treatment of Borderline Personality Disorder. New York, Guilford, 1993

Linehan MM, Armstrong HE, Suarez A, et al: Cognitive-behavioral treatment of chronically parasuicidal borderline patients. Arch Gen Psychiatry 48:1060–1064, 1991

Linehan MM, Dimeff LA, Reynolds SK, et al: Dialectical behavior therapy versus comprehensive validation therapy plus 12-step for the treatment of opioid dependent women meeting criteria for borderline personality disorder. Drug Alcohol Depend 67:13–26, 2002

Marlatt GA, Gordon JR (eds): Relapse Prevention: Maintenance Strategies in the Treatment of Addictive Behaviors. New York, Guilford, 1985

McCullough JP: Psychotherapy for dysthymia: a naturalistic study of ten patients. J Nerv Ment Dis 179:734–740, 1991

McCullough JP Jr: Skills Training Manual for Diagnosing and Treating Chronic Depression: Cognitive Behavioral Analysis System of Psychotherapy. New York, Guilford, 2001

Metropolitan Life Insurance Company: 1983 Metropolitan Height and Weight Tables. New York, Metropolitan Life Insurance Company, 1983

Miller WR, Yahne CE, Moyers TB, et al: A randomized trial of methods to help clinicians learn motivational interviewing. J Consult Clin Psychol 72:1050–1062, 2004

Mitchell JE, Peterson CB: Cognitive-behavioral treatments of eating disorders, in American Psychiatric Press Review of Psychiatry, Vol 16. Edited by Dickstein LJ, Riba MB, Oldham JM. Washington, DC, American Psychiatric Press, 1997, pp 107–133

Mitchell JE, Pyle RL, Eckert ED, et al: A comparison study of antidepressants and structured intensive group psychotherapy in the treatment of bulimia nervosa. Arch Gen Psychiatry 47:149–157, 1990

Monti PM, Rohsenow DJ, Rubonis AV, et al: Cue exposure with coping skills treatment for male alcoholics: a preliminary investigation. J Consult Clin Psychol 61:1011–1019, 1993

Morin CM: Cognitive-behavioral approaches to the treatment of insomnia. J Clin Psychiatry 65 (suppl 16):33–40, 2004

Newman CF, Leahy RL, Beck AT, et al: Bipolar Disorder: A Cognitive Therapy Approach. New York, American Psychological Association, 2002

Palmer RL, Birchall H, Damani S, et al: A dialectical behavior therapy program for people with an eating disorder and borderline personality disorder—description and outcome. Int J Eat Disord 33:281–286, 2003

Paul GL, Lentz RJ: Psychosocial Treatment of Chronic Mental Patients. Cambridge, MA, Harvard University Press, 1977

Perris C: Cognitive Therapy With Schizophrenic Patients. New York, Guilford, 1989

Prochaska JO, DiClemente CC: The transtheoretical approach, in Handbook of Psychotherapy Integration. Edited by Norcross JC, Goldfried MR. New York, Basic Books, 1992, pp 301–334

Project MATCH Research Group: Matching alcoholism treatments to client heterogeneity: treatment main effects and matching effects on drinking during treatment. J Stud Alcohol 59:631–639, 1998

Ricca V, Mannucci E, Zucchi T, et al: Cognitive-behavioural therapy for bulimia nervosa and binge eating disorder: a review. Psychother Psychosom 69:287–295, 2000

Robins CJ, Chapman AL: Dialectical behavior therapy: current status, recent developments, and future directions. J Personal Disord 18:73–89, 2004

Rush AJ, Weissenburger JE: Melancholic symptom features and DSM-IV. Am J Psychiatry 151:489–498, 1994

Scott J, Wright JH: Cognitive therapy for chronic and severe mental disorders, in American Psychiatric Press Review of Psychiatry, Vol 16. Edited by Dickstein LJ, Riba MB, Oldham JM. Washington, DC, American Psychiatric Press, 1997, pp 135–170

Scott J, Garland A, Moorhead S: A pilot study of cognitive therapy in bipolar disorders. Psychol Med 31:459–467, 2001

Sensky T, Turkington D, Kingdon D, et al: A randomized controlled trial of cognitive-behavioral therapy for persistent symptoms in schizophrenia resistant to medication. Arch Gen Psychiatry 57:165–172, 2000

Shea MT, Pilkonis PA, Beckham E, et al: Personality disorders and treatment outcome in the NIMH Treatment of Depression Collaborative Research Program. Am J Psychiatry 147:711–718, 1990

Strang J, McCambridge J: Can the practitioner correctly predict outcome in motivational interviewing? J Subst Abuse Treat 27:83–88, 2004

Stuart S, Simons AD, Thase ME, et al: Are personality assessments valid in acute major depression? J Affect Disord 24:281–290, 1992

Taylor HL, Keys A: Adaptation to caloric restriction. Science 112:215–218, 1950

Thase ME: The role of Axis II comorbidity in the management of patients with treatment-resistant depression. Psychiatr Clin North Am 19:287–309, 1996

Thase ME: Cognitive-behavioral therapy for substance abuse, in American Psychiatric Press Review of Psychiatry, Vol 16. Edited by Dickstein LJ, Riba MB, Oldham JM. Washington, DC, American Psychiatric Press, 1997, pp 45–71

Thase ME: The role of psychotherapy in the management of bipolar disorder, in Handbook of Bipolar Disorder. Edited by Kasper S, Hirschfeld RMA. New York, Marcel Dekker (in press)

Thase ME, Friedman ES: Is psychotherapy an effective treatment for melancholia and other severe depressive states? J Affect Disord 54:1–19, 1999

Thase ME, Howland R: Refractory depression: relevance of psychosocial factors and therapies. Psychiatr Ann 24:232–240, 1994

Thase ME, Wright JH: Cognitive behavior therapy manual for depressed inpatients: a treatment protocol outline. Behav Ther 22:579–595, 1991

Thase ME, Simons AD, Cahalane J, et al: Severity of depression and response to cognitive behavior therapy. Am J Psychiatry 148:784–789, 1991

Thase ME, Greenhouse JB, Frank E, et al: Treatment of major depression with psychotherapy or psychotherapy-pharmacotherapy combinations. Arch Gen Psychiatry 54:1009–1015, 1997

Turkington D, Dudley R, Warman DM, et al: Cognitive-behavioral therapy for schizophrenia: a review. J Psychiatr Pract 10:5–16, 2004

Walsh BT, Wilson GT, Loeb KL, et al: Medication and psychotherapy in the treatment of bulimia nervosa. Am J Psychiatry 154:523–531, 1997

Wilson GT: Cognitive behavior therapy for eating disorders: progress and problems. Behav Res Ther 37 (suppl 1):S79–S95, 1999

Woody GE, Munoz A: Efficacy, individual effectiveness, and population effectiveness in substance abuse treatment. Curr Psychiatry Rep 2:505–507, 2000

Woody GE, McLellan AT, Luborsky L: Psychiatric severity as a predictor of benefits from psychotherapy. Am J Psychiatry 141:1171–1177, 1984

Wright JH: Cognitive-behavior therapy for chronic depression. Psychiatr Ann 33:777–784, 2003

Wright JH, Thase ME, Beck AT, et al: Cognitive Therapy With Inpatients: Developing a Cognitive Milieu. New York, Guilford, 1993

Young J: Cognitive Therapy for Personality Disorders: A Schema-Focused Approach. Sarasota, FL, Professional Resource Exchange, 1990

11

Building Competence in Cognitive-Behavior Therapy

This volume is part of a series of books, Core Competencies in Psychotherapy (Glen O. Gabbard, M.D., series editor), devoted to helping readers achieve competence in delivering basic psychotherapies. The creation of the series was prompted in part by the American Association of Directors of Psychiatric Residency Training (AADPRT) adopting a policy of setting competency requirements in several core psychotherapies—including cognitive-behavior therapy (CBT) and psychodynamic therapy—for graduates of American psychiatry residency programs. So far in this book on CBT, we have not focused specifically on these competencies but have tried to provide information on the fundamentals of theory and technique that are needed to become a skilled cognitive-behavior therapist. In this last chapter, we detail the competency guidelines recommended by AADPRT, outline methods of measuring your progress in learning CBT, and suggest some ways to continue your development as a therapist.

Items mentioned in this chapter that are available in Appendix 1, "Worksheets and Checklists," are also available as a free download in larger format on the American Psychiatric Publishing Web site: http://www.appi.org/pdf/wright.

Core Competencies in CBT

The AADPRT competency standards for psychiatry residents (Sudak et al. 2001) are summarized in Table 11–1 (and are also available on the AADPRT Web site, http://www.aadprt.org). These standards are quite broad and should be useful to educators and trainees in CBT from a variety of disciplines. The competencies are grouped into three categories: knowledge, skills, and attitudes. When you review this list, you'll see that the standards are directly tied to the concepts and methods described in this book.

The main value of the AADPRT competency standards is in laying out specific goals for learning this form of therapy. If you have read the previous 10 chapters of this book, have had a basic course in CBT, and have been receiving feedback or supervision on your clinical skills, you should be in a good position to meet the AADPRT recommendations for competency. To get a sense of where you are in your path to learning CBT, we suggest that you perform the next learning exercise.

> **Learning Exercise 11–1.**   Self-Assessment of Competence in CBT
>
> 1. Review each item in Table 11–1.
>
> 2. Assess your knowledge, skills, and attitudes in CBT by giving yourself a score of excellent (E), satisfactory (S), or unsatisfactory (U) for each item. The standard for your self-assessment should not be at the master therapist level but at the level of a clinician who has completed residency courses, graduate training programs, or other concentrated educational programs in CBT.
>
> 3. If you noted problems in knowledge, skills, or attitudes for any items, think of a plan to upgrade your competence. Ideas might include rereading sections of this book, reviewing class notes, getting additional supervision, or studying other materials.

Table 11–1. Competency standards for cognitive-behavior therapy (CBT)

Knowledge	Skills	Attitudes
The clinician will demonstrate an understanding of	*The clinician will be able to*	*The clinician will be*
1. The cognitive-behavioral model.	1. Assess and conceptualize patients with the CBT model.	1. Empathic, respectful, nonjudgmental, and collaborative.
2. Concepts of automatic thoughts, cognitive errors, schemas, and behavioral principles.	2. Establish and maintain a collaborative therapeutic relationship.	2. Sensitive to sociocultural, socioeconomic, and educational issues.
3. Cognitive-behavioral formulations for common disorders.	3. Educate the patient about the CBT model.	3. Open to review of audio- or videotapes or direct observations of treatment sessions.
4. Indications for CBT.	4. Educate the patient about schemas and help him or her understand the origin of these beliefs.	
5. Rationale for structuring sessions, collaboration, and problem solving.	5. Structure sessions, including setting agendas, reviewing and assigning homework, working on key problems, and using feedback.	
6. Basic principles for psychoeducation.	6. Utilize activity scheduling and graded task assignments.	
7. Basic principles for behavioral methods.	7. Utilize relaxation training and graded exposure techniques.	
8. Basic principles for cognitive techniques such as modifying automatic thoughts and schemas.	8. Employ thought recording techniques.	
9. The importance of continued education in CBT.	9. Use relapse prevention techniques.	

Table 11–1. Competency standards for cognitive-behavior therapy (CBT) *(continued)*

Knowledge	Skills	Attitudes
	_____ 10. Recognize his or her own thoughts and feelings stimulated by the therapy.	
	_____ 11. Write a CBT formulation.	
	_____ 12. Seek appropriate consultation when needed.	

Source. Adapted from Sudak DM, Wright JH, Beck JS, et al: "AADPRT Cognitive Behavioral Therapy Competencies." Farmington, CT, American Association of Directors of Psychiatric Residency Training, 2001. Available at: http://www.aadprt.org. Accessed May 16, 2005.

Becoming a Competent Cognitive-Behavior Therapist

Although there are no published recommendations for standardized training in CBT, most experienced educators in this form of psychotherapy believe that a combination of learning experiences is required. For graduate students, residents, or other clinicians in training, these experiences usually include 1) a basic course (the Academy of Cognitive Therapy [ACT] recommends at least 40 hours of course work); 2) assigned readings (at least a core text on CBT theory and methods, such as this book and other targeted readings for special topics); 3) written case formulations; 4) case supervision (either in individual or group format, or both); 5) use of videotaped or audiotaped sessions that are reviewed and rated by an experienced cognitive-behavior therapist; and 6) significant practice in treating patients with CBT (treatment of 10 cases or more with varied diagnoses, including depression and different types of anxiety disorders).

A number of options are available for clinicians who completed their residency or graduate training programs before courses in CBT were offered or who believe that they need additional education to become skilled in CBT. The most rigorous and well-established training program for practicing clinicians is the fellowship at the Beck Institute in Philadelphia, Pennsylvania (http://www.beckinstitute.org). On-site fellowships and extramural fellowships are available. In each of these programs, the clinician receives extensive didactic instruction over at least a 6-month period, in addition to weekly individual supervision. For extramural fellows, the supervision is provided by telephone after the supervisor has reviewed tapes of the trainee's therapy sessions. Other centers for cognitive therapy also offer basic and advanced courses and supervision in individual or group settings (see Appendix 2, "Cognitive-Behavior Therapy Resources," for a listing of these centers).

An alternative method for training practicing clinicians is for an organization or agency to arrange a customized educational program. For example, one of us (J.H.W.) developed a yearlong curriculum for therapists at a large community mental health center. None of the clinicians attending the program had had any substantive prior training in CBT. As part of the program, four senior therapists enrolled in the extramural fellowship at the Beck Institute and then became assistants to the author in conducting the training for a group of more than 40 clinicians. The kickoff session for this training was an 8-hour workshop conducted by the author and Judith Beck, Ph.D., from the Beck Institute. This workshop was followed by weekly classes taught by the author, four additional intensive workshops, and weekly supervision provided by the extramural fellows. By the end of this year of training, the extramural fellows were able to continue the education of the other therapists at the agency by providing ongoing case supervision. Although significant resources were required to implement this training program, it was successful in educating a large number of clinicians in CBT.

Other practicing clinicians have obtained basic competence in CBT by participating in workshops at major scientific meetings, viewing videotapes of master therapists, attending retreats or camps designed to teach CBT (e.g., Camp Cognitive Therapy and other training workshops taught by Christine Padesky, Ph.D., and associates, http://www.padesky.com), and obtaining individual supervision in CBT (see Appendix 2, "Cognitive-Behavior Therapy Resources"). The Web site for the ACT (http://www.academyofct.org), a certifying organization in CBT, lists educational opportunities and provides a list of certified cognitive-behavior therapists who may be able to provide supervision or other training.

Measuring Your Progress

The CBT community is noted for having a long tradition of assessing the skills of clinicians and providing constructive feedback. Several rating scales, checklists, and tests are available (Sudak et al. 2003). Here we describe four instruments that you may find helpful for evaluating your progress in learning CBT.

Cognitive Therapy Scale

The principal measure used to give feedback on proficiency in CBT is the Cognitive Therapy Scale (CTS; see this chapter's appendix), developed by Young and Beck 1980 (Vallis et al. 1986). The CTS contains 11 items (e.g., agenda setting and structuring, collaboration, pacing and efficient use of time, guided discovery, focusing on key cognitions and behaviors, skill in applying CBT techniques, and homework) that are used to rate a therapist's performance on critical functions of CBT. Up to 6 points are awarded for each item on the CTS, thus yielding a maximum score of 66. An overall score of 40 is typically considered to represent satisfactory performance in CBT. The ACT requires that applicants for certification achieve a score of at least 40 on CTS ratings of a videotaped interview. In addition, a score of 40 on the CTS is commonly used as a measure for qualifying as a cognitive-behavior therapist for research investigations that study the effectiveness of this approach (Wright et al. 2005).

The CTS can help you learn about your strengths and weaknesses in doing CBT and can stimulate ideas for making improvements. In the next learning exercise, you are asked to rate one of your sessions on the CTS and to discuss these ratings with a colleague or supervisor.

> **Learning Exercise 11–2.** Using the Cognitive Therapy Scale
>
> 1. Record one of your CBT sessions on videotape or audiotape. This session should preferably be with an actual patient. However, a role-play session can also be used for this exercise.
>
> 2. Perform a self-rating on this session using the CTS. Also ask a supervisor or a colleague to rate the session.
>
> 3. Discuss the ratings with your supervisor or colleague.
>
> 4. Identify some of your strengths in the session.
>
> 5. If you or your colleague or supervisor identified any areas where you could improve your performance, list ideas you have for doing things differently.
>
> 6. Perform further ratings of videotaped or audiotaped sessions on a regular basis until you can routinely score 40 or above on this scale.

Cognitive Formulation Rating Scale

The ACT has developed specific guidelines for writing case conceptualizations to meet their criteria for certification in CBT. Detailed instructions for formulating cases and planning treatment can be found at the ACT Web site (http://www.academyofct.org). An example of a written case formulation also is provided on the Web site. A number of training programs in CBT have adopted the ACT guidelines and scoring system for case conceptualizations and require completion of one or more written formulations.

The system for formulating cases that we present in Chapter 3, "Assessment and Formulation," is based directly on the ACT guidelines.

Therefore, you should already know the basics of developing case conceptualizations that meet ACT standards. Ratings of components of the case conceptualization are made on a scale of 0–2 (0=not present, 1=present but inadequate, 2=present and adequate). Three general areas of performance are scored in the Cognitive Formulation Rating Scale (CFRS): 1) case history (two items), 2) formulation (five items), and 3) treatment plan and course of therapy (five items). The ACT standard for a passing score is 20 out of a possible 24 points. The scoring criteria for this scale are available on the ACT Web site.

We have found that writing out case formulations is one of the most worthwhile exercises for learning CBT. If you take the time to carefully think through formulations, commit them to paper, and get feedback from supervisors or other experienced cognitive-behavior therapists, you can build considerable sophistication and skill in this treatment approach. Although writing conceptualizations takes some effort, the rewards can be great.

> **Learning Exercise 11–3.** Using the
> Cognitive Formulation Rating Scale
>
> 1. Download the instructions for writing a case
>   conceptualization from the ACT Web site
>   (http://www.academyofct.org). Also review
>   the example of a written formulation and the
>   scoring criteria provided on the Web site.
>
> 2. Use the case formulation worksheet to
>   organize your key observations and plans.[1]
>   Then follow the ACT guidelines to write a full
>   case conceptualization.
>
> 3. Use the CFRS scoring criteria to perform a self-
>   rating of your written case conceptualization.
>
> 4. Ask a supervisor or experienced cognitive-
>   behavior therapist to score your
>   conceptualization and to discuss your ideas for
>   understanding and treating this case.

---

[1]For a blank copy of the worksheet, see Appendix 1, "Worksheets and Checklists." For more information about the worksheet, see Chapter 3, "Assessment and Formulation."

Cognitive Therapy Awareness Scale

Although the Cognitive Therapy Awareness Scale (CTAS) was originally developed to assess knowledge of CBT principles in patients treated with this form of therapy (Wright et al. 2002), it has subsequently been used in training programs as a pre- and posttest of awareness of basic concepts and terms. The CTAS is not a comprehensive measure of CBT knowledge, but it can be used to gauge progress in learning about key theories and methods. The scale includes 40 true-or-false questions on topics such as automatic thoughts, cognitive errors, schemas, thought recording, activity scheduling, and identifying cognitive distortions.

One point is awarded for each correct response to the 40 questions in the CTAS. Thus, a score of about 20 might be expected if the person taking the test had no prior knowledge of CBT. The maximum score on this scale is 40. Studies of the CTAS in patient populations have shown significant increases in scores after treatment with CBT (Wright et al. 2002, 2005). For example, in an investigation of 96 patients who received computer-assisted CBT for depression or anxiety, mean scores improved from 24.2 before treatment to 32.5 after using the computer program (Wright et al. 2002). Although the CTAS has not been studied formally in training applications, our experience in using this scale with psychiatry residents suggests that mean scores before a basic course in CBT typically range from the mid-20s to the lower 30s. As expected, CTAS scores usually increase substantially after completing course work, readings, and other educational experiences in CBT. The CTAS is published in Wright et al. 2002.

Cognitive-Behavior Therapy Supervision Checklist

If you are receiving or providing supervision in CBT, you may be interested in using the Cognitive-Behavior Therapy Supervision Checklist, a form developed by several members of the AADPRT competency standards work group (Sudak et al. 2001). This checklist is divided into two sections: 1) competencies that should be demonstrated in each session (e.g., "maintains collaborative-empirical alliance," "demonstrates ability to use guided discovery," and "effectively sets agenda and structures session"), and 2) competencies that may be demonstrated over a course of therapy or therapies (e.g., "sets goals and plans treatment based on CBT formulation," "educates patient about CBT model and/or therapy interventions," and "can utilize activity or pleasant events scheduling"). The Cognitive-Behavior Therapy Supervision Checklist is available in Appendix 1, "Worksheets and Checklists."

Continued Experience and Training in CBT

To retain your skills in CBT, it will be important to practice cognitive-behavioral interventions regularly and to take advantage of postgraduate education opportunities. Also, if you wish to add depth and range to your abilities, you will need to explore options for further learning. Our experiences in training and supervising clinicians in CBT suggest that skills can atrophy if they are not used regularly and stimulated by ongoing educational activities.

Earlier in this chapter, we suggested that attending workshops at scientific meetings, viewing videotapes of accomplished cognitive-behavior therapists, and going to educational retreats or camps can be used to build basic competency (see "Becoming a Competent Cognitive-Behavior Therapist"). These same experiences can play a useful role in helping clinicians maintain their CBT skills and develop new areas of expertise. For example, courses or workshops on CBT methods for bipolar disorder, treatment-resistant depression, schizophrenia, eating disorders, posttraumatic stress disorder, chronic pain, personality disorders, and other conditions are commonly offered at national and international conferences (e.g., annual meetings of the American Psychiatric Association, the American Psychological Association, and the Association for Advancement of Behavior Therapy; see Appendix 2, "Cognitive-Behavior Therapy Resources").

Readings in CBT also can help you learn new ways to apply these methods. A list of books that can expand your knowledge of CBT is provided in Appendix 2, "Cognitive-Behavior Therapy Resources." We have included classic texts such as those by A. T. Beck and colleagues on depression, anxiety disorders, and personality disorders, in addition to volumes on diverse topics such as marital and group therapies, treatment of psychosis, and advanced CBT techniques.

Another way to work on improving CBT proficiency is to apply for certification from the ACT (http://www.academyofct.org). Some of the certification criteria for this organization, including submission of videotaped material for rating on the CTS and writing a case formulation that follows the ACT guidelines, are discussed earlier in this chapter (see sections "Cognitive Therapy Scale" and "Cognitive Formulation Rating Scale"). Studying and preparing for an ACT certification submission can be a valuable tactic for sharpening your ability to perform CBT. Certified members of the ACT also have access to a number of superb continuing-education opportunities, including subscribing to e-mail communications lists, receiving updates on new developments in CBT, and attending special lectures by leading clinicians and researchers.

Our final suggestion for continuing your growth as a cognitive-behavior therapist is to attend an ongoing seminar or CBT supervision group. These types of group learning experiences are offered routinely at CBT centers, educational institutions, and other clinical and research settings. The weekly supervision group in the principal author's clinic offers reviews and ratings of videotaped sessions, role-play demonstrations, and learning modules designed to help clinicians expand their abilities in specific CBT applications (e.g., treatment-resistant depression, personality disorders, inpatient CBT, group therapy, and fibromyalgia). Although the level of experience in CBT typically ranges from novice to expert, responsibility for bringing material to meetings and contributing to the educational process nevertheless rotates among all participants. If you do not have a similar group available in your community, you might consider starting one. Many cognitive-behavior therapists highly value these ongoing supervision groups because they provide a stimulating and collegial forum for learning.

Summary

In this concluding chapter, we described several useful ways of assessing proficiency and suggested methods for expanding knowledge and building expertise. Efforts to continue developing skills in this therapy approach can have many benefits. Being able to deliver treatment competently and consistently should help you achieve good results. In addition, specific CBT methods are now available for virtually all psychiatric disorders for which psychotherapy is indicated. Studying these methods can help you increase your abilities to treat diverse groups of patients effectively. We hope that further education in this form of therapy will give you a deeper understanding of the cognitive-behavioral paradigm and its power to change patients' lives.

References

Sudak DM, Wright JH, Beck JS, et al: AADPRT Cognitive Behavioral Therapy Competencies. Farmington, CT, American Association of Directors of Psychiatric Residency Training, 2001. Available at: http://www.aadprt.org. Accessed May 16, 2005.

Sudak DM, Beck JS, Wright JH: Cognitive behavioral therapy: a blueprint for attaining and assessing psychiatry resident competency. Acad Psychiatry 27:154–159, 2003

Vallis TM, Shaw BF, Dobson KS: The Cognitive Therapy Scale: psychometric properties. J Consult Clin Psychol 54:381–385, 1986

Wright JH, Wright AS, Salmon P, et al: Development and initial testing of a multimedia program for computer-assisted cognitive therapy. Am J Psychother 56:76–86, 2002

Wright JH, Wright AS, Albano AM, et al: Computer-assisted cognitive therapy for depression: maintaining efficacy while reducing therapist time. Am J Psychiatry 162:1158–1164, 2005

Young J, Beck AT: Cognitive Therapy Scale Rating Manual. Philadelphia, PA, Center for Cognitive Therapy, 1980

Appendix:
Cognitive Therapy Scale

Therapist: _____   Patient: _____

Date of Session:_____   Session No.: _____

Directions: Rate performance on a scale from 0 to 6, and record the rating on the line next to the item number. Descriptions are provided for even-numbered scale points. If you believe the rating falls between two of the descriptors, select the intervening odd number (1, 3, 5).

   If the descriptions for an item occasionally do not seem to apply to the session you are rating, feel free to disregard them and use the more general scale below:

0	1	2	3	4	5	6
Poor	Barely adequate	Mediocre	Satisfactory	Good	Very good	Excellent

Part I. General Therapeutic Skills

___1. Agenda

0 Therapist did not set agenda.

2 Therapist set agenda that was vague or incomplete.

4 Therapist worked with patient to set a mutually satisfactory agenda that included specific target problems (e.g., anxiety at work, dissatisfaction with marriage).

6 Therapist worked with patient to set an appropriate agenda with target problems, suitable for the available time. Established priorities and then followed agenda.

___2. Feedback

0 Therapist did not ask for feedback to determine the patient's understanding of, or response to, the session.

2 Therapist elicited some feedback from the patient but did not ask enough questions to be sure the patient understood the therapist's line of reasoning during the session or to ascertain whether the patient was satisfied with the session.

Source.   Reprinted from Young JE, Beck AT: Cognitive Therapy Scale. Philadelphia, University of Pennsylvania, 1980. Used with permission.

4   Therapist asked enough questions to be sure that the patient understood the therapist's line of reasoning throughout the session and to determine the patient's reactions to the session. The therapist adjusted his or her behavior in response to the feedback, when appropriate.

6   Therapist was especially adept at eliciting and responding to verbal and nonverbal feedback throughout the session (e.g., elicited reactions to session, regularly checked for understanding, helped summarize main points at end of session).

___3. Understanding

0   Therapist repeatedly failed to understand what the patient explicitly said and thus consistently missed the point. Poor empathic skills.

2   Therapist was usually able to reflect or rephrase what the patient explicitly said, but repeatedly failed to respond to more subtle communication. Limited ability to listen and empathize.

4   Therapist generally seemed to grasp the patient's "internal reality" as reflected by both what was explicitly said and what the patient communicated in more subtle ways. Good ability to listen and empathize.

6   Therapist seemed to understand the patient's "internal reality" thoroughly and was adept at communicating this understanding through appropriate verbal and nonverbal responses to the patient (e.g., the tone of the therapist's response conveyed a sympathetic understanding of the patient's "message"). Excellent listening and empathic skills.

___4. Interpersonal Effectiveness

0   Therapist had poor interpersonal skills. Seemed hostile, demeaning, or in some other way destructive to the patient.

2   Therapist did not seem destructive but had significant interpersonal problems. At times, therapist appeared unnecessarily impatient, aloof, or insincere or had difficulty conveying confidence and competence.

4   Therapist displayed a satisfactory degree of warmth, concern, confidence, genuineness, and professionalism. No significant interpersonal problems.

6   Therapist displayed optimal levels of warmth, concern, confidence, genuineness, and professionalism, appropriate for this particular patient in this session.

___5. Collaboration

0   Therapist did not attempt to set up a collaboration with the patient.
2   Therapist attempted to collaborate with the patient but had difficulty either defining a problem that the patient considered important or establishing rapport.
4   Therapist was able to collaborate with the patient, focus on a problem that both the patient and therapist considered important, and establish rapport.
6   Collaboration seemed excellent; the therapist encouraged the patient as much as possible to take an active role during the session (e.g., by offering choices) so they could function as a team.

___6. Pacing and Efficient Use of Time

0   Therapist made no attempt to structure therapy time. Session seemed aimless.
2   Session had some direction, but the therapist had significant problems with structuring or pacing (e.g., too little structure, inflexible about structure, too slowly paced, too rapidly paced).
4   Therapist was reasonably successful at using time efficiently. Therapist maintained appropriate control over flow of discussion and pacing.
6   Therapist used time efficiently by tactfully limiting peripheral and unproductive discussion and by pacing the session as rapidly as was appropriate for the patient.

Part II. Conceptualization, Strategy, and Technique

___7. Guided Discovery

0   Therapist relied primarily on debate, persuasion, or "lecturing." Therapist seemed to be cross-examining the patient, putting the patient on the defensive, or forcing his or her point of view on the patient.
2   Therapist relied too heavily on persuasion and debate, rather than guided discovery. However, therapist's style was supportive enough that patient did not seem to feel attacked or defensive.
4   Therapist, for the most part, helped the patient see new perspectives through guided discovery (e.g., examining evidence, considering alternatives, weighing advantages and disadvantages) rather than through debate. Used questioning appropriately.

6   Therapist was especially adept at using guided discovery during the session to explore problems and help the patient draw his or her own conclusions. Achieved an excellent balance between skillful questioning and other modes of intervention.

___8. Focusing on Key Cognitions or Behaviors

0   Therapist did not attempt to elicit specific thoughts, assumptions, images, meanings, or behaviors.

2   Therapist used appropriate techniques to elicit cognitions or behaviors; however, the therapist had difficulty finding a focus, or focused on cognitions and behaviors that were irrelevant to the patient's key problems.

4   Therapist focused on specific cognitions or behaviors relevant to the target problem. However, the therapist could have focused on more central cognitions or behaviors that offered greater promise for progress.

6   Therapist very skillfully focused on key thoughts, assumptions, behaviors, etc., that were most relevant to the problem area and offered considerable promise for progress.

___9. Strategy for Change

(*Note:* For this item, focus on the quality of the therapist's strategy for change, not on how effectively the strategy was implemented or whether change actually occurred.)

0   Therapist did not select cognitive-behavioral techniques.

2   Therapist selected cognitive-behavioral techniques; however, the overall strategy for bringing about change either seemed vague or did not seem promising in helping the patient.

4   Therapist seemed to have a generally coherent strategy for change that showed reasonable promise and incorporated cognitive-behavioral techniques.

6   Therapist followed a consistent strategy for change that seemed very promising, and incorporated the most appropriate cognitive-behavioral techniques.

___10. Application of Cognitive-Behavioral Techniques

(*Note:* For this item, focus on how skillfully the techniques were applied, not on how appropriate they were for the target problem or whether change actually occurred.)

0   Therapist did not apply any cognitive-behavioral techniques.
2   Therapist used cognitive-behavioral techniques, but there were significant flaws in the way they were applied.
4   Therapist applied cognitive-behavioral techniques with moderate skill.
6   Therapist very skillfully and resourcefully employed cognitive-behavioral techniques.

___11. Homework

0   Therapist did not attempt to incorporate homework relevant to cognitive therapy.
2   Therapist had significant difficulties incorporating homework (e.g., did not review previous homework, did not explain homework in sufficient detail, assigned inappropriate homework).
4   Therapist reviewed previous homework and assigned "standard" cognitive therapy homework generally relevant to issues dealt with in session. Homework was explained in sufficient detail.
6   Therapist reviewed previous homework and carefully assigned homework drawn from cognitive therapy for the coming week. Assignment seemed custom-tailored to help patient incorporate new perspectives, test hypotheses, experiment with new behaviors discussed during session, etc.

___Total Score

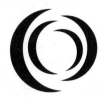

Appendix 1

Worksheets and Checklists

Contents

Appendix 1 is available as a free download in its entirety and in larger format on the American Psychiatric Publishing Web site: http://www.appi.org/pdf/wright.
[a]Adapted with permission from Wright JH, Wright AS, Beck AT: *Good Days Ahead: The Multimedia Program for Cognitive Therapy*. Louisville, KY, Mindstreet, 2004. Permission is granted for readers to use these items in clinical practice.

Cognitive-Behavior Therapy
Case Formulation Worksheet

Patient Name:	Date:	
Diagnoses/Symptoms:		
Formative Influences:		
Situational Issues:		
Biological, Genetic, and Medical Factors:		
Strengths/Assets:		
Treatment Goals:		

Event 1	Event 2	Event 3
Automatic Thoughts	Automatic Thoughts	Automatic Thoughts
Emotions	Emotions	Emotions
Behaviors	Behaviors	Behaviors

Schemas:
Working Hypothesis:
Treatment Plan:

Note. Available at: http://www.appi.org/pdf/wright.

Automatic Thoughts Checklist

Instructions: Place a check mark beside each negative automatic thought that you have had in the past 2 weeks.

_____ I should be doing better in life.

_____ He/she doesn't understand me.

_____ I've let him/her down.

_____ I just can't enjoy things anymore.

_____ Why am I so weak?

_____ I always keep messing things up.

_____ My life's going nowhere.

_____ I can't handle it.

_____ I'm failing.

_____ It's too much for me.

_____ I don't have much of a future.

_____ Things are out of control.

_____ I feel like giving up.

_____ Something bad is sure to happen.

_____ There must be something wrong with me.

Note. Available at: http://www.appi.org/pdf/wright.

Thought Change Record

Situation	Automatic thought(s)	Emotion(s)	Rational response	Outcome
Describe a. Actual event leading to unpleasant emotion *or* b. Stream of thoughts leading to unpleasant emotion *or* c. Unpleasant physiological sensations.	a. *Write* automatic thought(s) that preceded emotion(s). b. *Rate* belief in automatic thought(s), 0%–100%.	a. *Specify* sad, anxious, angry, etc. b. *Rate* degree of emotion, 1%–100%.	a. *Identify* cognitive errors. b. *Write* rational response to automatic thought(s). c. *Rate* belief in rational response, 0%–100%.	a. *Specify and rate* subsequent emotion(s), 0%–100%. b. *Describe* changes in behavior.

Note. Available at: http://www.appi.org/pdf/wright.

Source. Adapted from Beck AT, Rush AJ, Shaw BF, et al: *Cognitive Therapy of Depression.* New York, Guilford, 1979, pp. 164–165. Used with permission.

Definitions of Cognitive Errors

Selective abstraction (sometimes called *ignoring the evidence* or *the mental filter*) A conclusion is drawn after looking at only a small portion of the available information. Salient data are screened out or ignored in order to confirm the person's biased view of the situation.

> *Example:* A depressed man with low self-esteem doesn't receive a holiday card from an old friend. He thinks, "I'm losing all my friends; nobody cares about me anymore." He is ignoring the evidence that he has received a number of other cards, his old friend has sent him a card every year for the past 15 years, his friend has been busy this past year with a move and a new job, and he still has good relationships with other friends.

Arbitrary inference Coming to a conclusion in the face of contradictory evidence or in the absence of evidence.

> *Example:* A woman with fear of elevators is asked to predict the chances that an elevator will fall if she rides in it. She replies that the chances are 10% or more that the elevator will fall to the ground and she will be injured. Many people have tried to convince her that the chances of a catastrophic elevator accident are negligible.

Overgeneralization A conclusion is made about one or more isolated incidents and then is extended illogically to cover broad areas of functioning.

> *Example:* A depressed college student gets a B on a test. He considers this unsatisfactory. He overgeneralizes when he has these automatic thoughts: "I'm in trouble in this class....I'm falling short everywhere in my life....I can't do anything right."

Magnification and minimization The significance of an attribute, event, or sensation is exaggerated or minimized.

> *Example:* A woman with panic disorder starts to feel light-headed during the onset of a panic attack. She thinks, "I'll faint....I might have a heart attack or a stroke."

Personalization External events are related to oneself when there is little evidence for doing so. Excessive responsibility or blame is taken for negative events.

Example: There has been an economic downturn, and a previously successful business is now struggling to meet the annual budget. Layoffs are being considered. A host of factors have led to the budget crisis, but one of the managers thinks, "It's all my fault....I should have seen this coming and done something about it....I've failed everyone in the company."

Dichotomous thinking (also called *absolutistic thinking* or *all-or-nothing thinking*) Judgments about oneself, personal experiences, or others are placed into one of two categories: all bad or all good; total failure or complete success; completely flawed or absolutely perfect.

Example: David, a man with depression, compares himself with Ted, a friend who appears to have a good marriage and whose children are doing well in school. Although the friend has a fair amount of domestic happiness, his life is far from ideal. Ted has troubles at work, financial strains, and physical ailments, among other difficulties. David is engaging in absolutistic thinking when he tells himself, "Ted has everything going for him....I have nothing."

Examining the Evidence for Automatic Thoughts Worksheet

Instructions:

1. Identify a negative or troubling automatic thought.
2. Then list all the evidence that you can find that either supports ("evidence for") or disproves ("evidence against") the automatic thought.
3. After trying to find cognitive errors in the "evidence for" column, you can write revised or alternative thoughts at the bottom of the page.

Automatic thought:

Evidence for automatic thought:

1.

2.

3.

4.

5.

Evidence against automatic thought:

1.

2.

3.

4.

5.

Cognitive errors:

Alternative thoughts:

Note. Available at: http://www.appi.org/pdf/wright.

Weekly Activity Schedule

Instructions: Write down your activities for each hour and then rate them on a scale of 0–10 for mastery (**m**) or degree of accomplishment and for pleasure (**p**) or amount of enjoyment you experienced. A rating of 0 would mean that you had no sense of mastery or pleasure. A rating of 10 would mean that you experienced maximum mastery or pleasure.

	Sunday	Monday	Tuesday	Wednesday	Thursday	Friday	Saturday
8:00 A.M.							
9:00 A.M.							
10:00 A.M.							
11:00 A.M.							
12:00 P.M.							
1:00 P.M.							
2:00 P.M.							
3:00 P.M.							
4:00 P.M.							
5:00 P.M.							
6:00 P.M.							
7:00 P.M.							
8:00 P.M.							
9:00 P.M.							

Note.   Available at: http://www.appi.org/pdf/wright.

Schema Inventory

Instructions: Use this checklist to search for possible underlying rules of thinking. Place a check mark beside each schema that you think you may have.

Healthy Schemas

___ No matter what happens, I can manage somehow.

___ If I work hard at something, I can master it.

___ I'm a survivor.

___ Others trust me.

___ I'm a solid person.

___ People respect me.

___ They can knock me down, but they can't knock me out.

___ I care about other people.

___ If I prepare in advance, I usually do better.

___ I deserve to be respected.

___ I like to be challenged.

___ There's not much that can scare me.

___ I'm intelligent.

___ I can figure things out.

___ I'm friendly.

___ I can handle stress.

___ The tougher the problem, the tougher I become.

___ I can learn from my mistakes and be a better person.

___ I'm a good spouse (and/or parent, child, friend, lover).

___ Everything will work out all right.

Dysfunctional Schemas

___ I must be perfect to be accepted.

___ If I choose to do something, I must succeed.

___ I'm stupid.

___ Without a woman (man), I'm nothing.

___ I'm a fake.

___ Never show weakness.

___ I'm unlovable.

___ If I make one mistake, I'll lose everything.

___ I'll never be comfortable around others.

___ I can never finish anything.

___ No matter what I do, I won't succeed.

___ The world is too frightening for me.

___ Others can't be trusted.

___ I must always be in control.

___ I'm unattractive.

___ Never show your emotions.

___ Other people will take advantage of me.

___ I'm lazy.

___ If people really knew me, they wouldn't like me.

___ To be accepted, I must always please others.

Note. Available at: http://www.appi.org/pdf/wright.

Examining the Evidence for Schemas Worksheet

Instructions:

1. Identify a negative or maladaptive schema that you would like to change, and write it down on this form.
2. Write down any evidence that either supports or disproves this schema.
3. Look for cognitive errors in the evidence for the maladaptive schema.
4. Finally, note your ideas for changing the schema and your plans for putting these ideas into action.

Schema I want to change:

Evidence for this schema:	**Evidence against this schema:**
1.	1.
2.	2.
3.	3.
4.	4.
5.	5.

Cognitive errors:

Now that I've examined the evidence, my degree of belief in the schema is:

Ideas I have for modifications to this schema:

Actions I will take now to change my schema and act in a healthier way:

Note.   Available at: http://www.appi.org/pdf/wright.

Cognitive-Behavior Therapy Supervision Checklist[a]

Therapist _____

Supervisor _____ Date _____

Instructions: Use this checklist to monitor and evaluate competencies in CBT. Listed in Part A are competencies that should typically be demonstrated in each session. Part B contains competencies that may be demonstrated over a course of therapy or therapies. The checklist is not intended for evaluation of performance in first or last sessions.

Part A: Competencies that should typically be demonstrated in each session.

Competency	Superior	Satisfactory	Needs improve-ment	Did not attempt or N/A
1. Maintains collaborative empirical alliance				
2. Expresses appropriate empathy, genuineness				
3. Demonstrates accurate understanding				
4. Maintains appropriate professionalism and boundaries				
5. Elicits and gives appropriate feedback				
6. Demonstrates knowledge of CBT model				
7. Demonstrates ability to use guided discovery				
8. Effectively sets agenda and structures session				
9. Reviews and assigns useful homework				
10. Identifies automatic thoughts and/or beliefs (schemas)				
11. Modifies automatic thoughts and/or beliefs (schemas)				

Note. Available at: http://www.appi.org/pdf/wright.

Competency	Superior	Satisfactory	Needs improve-ment	Did not attempt or N/A
12. Utilizes behavioral intervention or assists patient with problem solving				
13. Applies CBT methods in flexible manner that meets needs of patient				

Part B: Competencies that may be demonstrated over a course of therapy or therapies

Competency	Superior	Satisfactory	Needs improve-ment	Did not attempt or N/A
1. Sets goals and plans treatment based on CBT formulation				
2. Educates patient about CBT model and/or therapy interventions				
3. Demonstrates ability to use thought record or other structured method of responding to dysfunctional cognitions				
4. Can utilize activity or pleasant events scheduling				
5. Can utilize exposure and response prevention or graded task assignment				
6. Can utilize relaxation and/or stress management techniques				
7. Can utilize CBT relapse prevention methods				
Comments:				

[a]Checklist developed by Jesse H. Wright, M.D., Ph.D., Donna Sudak, M.D., David Bienenfeld, M.D., and Judith Beck, Ph.D., 2001.

Note. Available at: http://www.appi.org/pdf/wright.

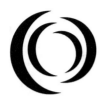

Appendix 2

Cognitive-Behavior Therapy Resources

Self-Help Books

Basco MR: Never Good Enough: How to Use Perfectionism to Your Advantage Without Letting It Ruin Your Life. New York, Free Press, 1999

Burns DD: Feeling Good: The New Mood Therapy, Revised Edition. New York, Avon, 1999

Craske MG, Barlow DH: Mastery of Your Anxiety and Panic, 3rd Edition. San Antonio, TX, Psychological Corporation, 2000

Foa EB, Wilson R: Stop Obsessing! How to Overcome Your Obsessions and Compulsions, Revised Edition. New York, Bantam, 2001

Greenberger D, Padesky CA: Mind Over Mood: Change How You Feel by Changing the Way You Think. New York, Guilford, 1996

Wright JH, Basco MR: Getting Your Life Back: The Complete Guide to Recovery From Depression. New York, Free Press, 2001

Computer Programs

FearFighter. Coventry, England, ST Solutions, 1996. Available at: http://fearfighter.com.

Tanner S, Ball J: Beating the Blues: A Self-Help Approach to Overcoming Depression. Randwick, Australia, Tanner and Ball, 1998. Available at: http://beatingtheblues.com.

Virtual reality programs by Rothbaum B et al. Decatur, GA, Virtually Better, 1996. Available at: http://virtuallybetter.com.

Wright JH, Wright AS, Beck AT: Good Days Ahead: The Multimedia Program for Cognitive Therapy. Louisville, KY, Mindstreet, 2004. Available at: http://www.mindstreet.com.

Videos of Master Cognitive-Behavior Therapists

Aaron T. Beck, M.D.: Demonstration of the Cognitive Therapy of Depression: Interview #1 (Patient With Family Problem). VHS or DVD. Bala Cynwyd, PA, Beck Institute for Cognitive Therapy and Research, 1977. Available from: http://beckinstitute.org.

Aaron T. Beck, M.D.: Cognitive Therapy of Depression: Interview #1 (Patient With Hopelessness Problem). VHS or DVD. Bala Cynwyd, PA, Beck Institute for Cognitive Therapy and Research, 1979. Available from: http://beckinstitute.org.

Judith S. Beck, Ph.D.: Brief Therapy Inside Out: Cognitive Therapy of Depression. VHS. Bala Cynwyd, PA, Beck Institute for Cognitive Therapy and Research, 1979. Available from: http://beckinstitute.org.

Arthur Freeman, Ed.D.: Cognitive-Behavioral Couples Therapy (Psychotherapy Videotape Series—IV, Relationships). VHS. Washington, DC, American Psychological Association, 2004. Available from: http://apa.org.

Donald Meichenbaum, Ph.D.: Cognitive-Behavioral Therapy With Donald Meichenbaum, Ph.D. VHS. New York, Insight Media, 2000. Available from: http://www.insight-media.com.

Christine Padesky, Ph.D.: Cognitive Therapy for Panic Disorder. VHS or DVD. Huntington Beach, CA, Center for Cognitive Therapy, 1993. Available from: http://padesky.com.

Christine Padesky, Ph.D.: Guided Discovery Using Socratic Dialogue. VHS or DVD. Huntington Beach, CA, Center for Cognitive Therapy, 1996. Available from: http://padesky.com.

Professional Organizations With Special Interest in Cognitive-Behavior Therapy

Academy of Cognitive Therapy (http://www.academyofct.org)

American Association of Directors of Psychiatric Residency Training (http://aadprt.org)

Association for Advancement of Behavior Therapy (http://www.aabt.org)

British Association for Behavioural and Cognitive Psychotherapies (http://www.babcp.com)

European Association for Behavioural and Cognitive Therapies (http://www.eabct.com)

French Association for Behaviour and Cognitive Therapy (Association Française de Thérapie Comportementale et Cognitive; http://www.aftcc.org)

International Association for Cognitive Psychotherapy (http://www.cognitivetherapyassociation.org)

Centers of Cognitive-Behavior Therapy

United States

Alabama. Alabama Center for Cognitive Therapy, 7 Huddle Drive, Suite C, Birmingham, AL 35243, Phone: (205) 967-6611

Arizona. Center for Cognitive Therapy, 6991 East Camelback, Suite B-302, Scottsdale, AZ 85251, Phone: (480) 949-7995

California.

Fremont. Center for Cognitive Therapy, 39025 Sandale Drive, Fremont, CA 34538

Huntington Beach. Center for Cognitive Therapy, P.O. Box 5308, Huntington Beach, CA 92615-5308, Phone: (714) 963-0528, E-mail: mooney@padesky.com; Web: http://www.padesky.com

La Jolla. La Jolla Center for Cognitive Therapy, 8950 Villa La Jolla Drive, Suite 1130, La Jolla, CA 92037, Phone: (858) 450-0460, E-mail: cwiese5256@cs.com, brendaj@adnc.com, ATHorvath@cs.com

Oakland. Center for Cognitive Therapy, 5435 College Avenue, Suite 102, Oakland, CA 94818-1502, Phone: (415) 652-4455

San Diego. Cognitive Therapy Institute, 3262 Holiday Court, Suite 220, La Jolla, CA 92037, Phone: (858) 450-1101, E-mail: Jimshenk2@cs.com

Colorado. Cognitive Therapy Center of Denver, 2055 S. Oneida Street, Suite 264, Denver, CO 80224, Phone: (303) 639-9337

District of Columbia. Washington Center for Cognitive Therapy, 5225 Connecticut Avenue NW, Suite 501, Washington, D.C. 20015, Phone: (202) 244-0260

Florida. Florida Center for Cognitive Therapy, 2753 State Road 580, Suite 103, Clearwater, FL 34627

Georgia. Atlanta Center for Cognitive Therapy, 1772 Century Blvd., Atlanta, GA 30345, Phone: (404) 248-1159 or (800) 789-2228 for training program for professionals, E-mail: acct@cognitiveatlanta.com; Web: http://www. cognitiveatlanta.com

Illinois.

Chicago. Center for Cognitive Therapy, Department of Psychiatry, Northwestern University Medical School, 222 East Superior Street, Suite 200, Chicago, IL 60611

Cognitive Behavior Therapy Program, Department of Psychiatry (MC 913), University of Illinois at Chicago, 912 S. Wood Street, Chicago, IL 60612

Cognitive Therapy Program, 1725 W. Harrison Street, Suite 958, Chicago, IL 60612, Phone: (312) 226-0300

Kentucky. Kentucky Center for Cognitive Therapy, University of Louisville School of Medicine, Norton Psychiatric Center, PO Box 35070, Louisville, KY 40232, Phone: (502) 629-8880, E-mail: jwright@iglou.com

Maryland.

Baltimore. Baltimore Center for Cognitive Therapy, 6303 Greenspring Avenue, Baltimore, MD 21209, Phone: (301) 365-5959

Chevy Chase. Cognitive Therapy Center, 5530 Wisconsin Avenue, Suite 915, Chevy Chase, MD 20815, Phone: (301) 951-3668

Bethesda. Washington DC Area Center for Cognitive Therapy, 6310 Winston Drive, Bethesda, MD 20817, Phone: (301) 229-3066

Massachusetts.

Boston. Cognitive Therapy Research Program, Bay Cove Bldg., Suite 550, 66 Canal Street, Boston, MA 02114, Phone: (617) 742-3939

Newton Centre. The Center for Cognitive Therapy, 10 Langley Road, Suite 200, Newton Centre, MA 02158, Phone: (617) 527-3041

New Jersey. Cognitive Therapy Center of New Jersey, 49 Maple Street, Suite 401, Summit, NJ 07901, Phone: (908) 227-1550

New York.

Albany. Center for Cognitive Therapy of the Capital District, One Pinnacle Place, Suite 207, Albany, NY 12203, Phone: (518) 482-1815, E-mail: Johnel@aol.com, Dr_DMcCarthy@aol.com

Brooklyn. Cognitive Therapy Center of Brooklyn, 207 Berkeley Place, Brooklyn, NY 11217, Phone: (718) 636-5071

Great Neck (on Long Island). Cognitive Therapy Center of Long Island, 11 Middle Neck Road, Suite 207, Great Neck, NY 11021, Phone: (516) 466-8485

New York. American Institute for Cognitive Therapy, 136 East 57th Street, Suite 1101, New York, NY 10022, Phone: (212) 308-2440, E-mail: AICT@AOL.com; Web: http://www.cognitivetherapynyc.com

Cognitive Therapy Center of New York, 3 East 80th Street, New York, NY 10021

Long Island Center for Cognitive Therapy, 31 East 12th Street, Suite 1E, New York, NY 10003, Phone: (212) 254-0294, Web: http://www.facethefear.com

Nyack. Hudson Valley Center for Cognitive Therapy, 99 Main Street, Suite 114, Nyack, NY 10960, Phone: (845) 353-3399

North Carolina. Center for Cognitive Therapy of North Carolina, 2412 Basil Drive, Raleigh, NC 27612-2874, Phone: (919) 676-6711, E-mail: comprehab @mindspring.com

Ohio.

Cleveland. Cleveland Center for Cognitive Therapy, 24400 Highpoint Road, Suite 9, Beachwood, OH 44122, Phone: (216) 831-2500, E-mail: jpretzer@apk.net; Web: http://www.behavioralhealthassoc.com

Columbus (with branches in Reynoldsburg and Mt. Vernon). Center for Cognitive and Behavioral Therapy of Greater Columbus, 2121 Bethel Road, Suites C and E, Columbus, OH 43220, Phone: (614) 459-4490, E-mail: kda1757@earthlink.net

Pennsylvania.

Philadelphia. Beck Institute for Cognitive Therapy and Research, 1 Belmont Avenue, Suite 700, Bala Cynwyd, PA 19004-1610, Phone: (610) 664-3020, E-mail:beckinst@gim.net; Web: http://www.beckinstitute.org

Center for Cognitive Therapy, University of Pennsylvania, Philadelphia, PA 19104, Phone: (215) 898-3466

Tennessee. Center for Cognitive Therapy, 340 21st Avenue North, Nashville, TN 37203, Phone: (615) 329-9057

Texas. Center for Cognitive Therapy, Glen Lakes Tower, 9400 N. Central Expressway, Suite 1212, Dallas, TX 75235, Phone: (214) 373-9605, E-mail: drpaul@why.net

Wisconsin. Cognitive Therapy Institute of Milwaukee, 1220 Dewey Avenue, Wauwatosa, WI 53213

Wyoming. Cognitive Therapy Program, 610 West Broadway, Suite L02B, Jackson, WY 83001, E-mail: Doctorjdoucette@aol.com

Australia

Centre for Cognitive Behaviour Therapy, 45 Balcombe Road, Mentone 3195, Melbourne, Australia, Phone: (03) 9585 1881; Web: http://www.ccbt.com.au

Brazil

Sociedade Brasileira de Terapias Cognitivas, Rua Jardim Botânico, 674—sala 108, Jardim Botânico, CEP: 22461-000, Rio de Janeiro, Brazil, Phone: (21) 2540-5238, E-mail: sbtc@sbtc.org.br; Web: http://www.sbtc.org.br

Canada

Toronto Center for Cognitive Therapy, Scotia Plaza, 49th Floor, 40 King Street West, Toronto, ON M5H 4A2, Canada, Phone: (416) 777-6699, E-mail: dubord@aol.com

United Kingdom

Oxford Cognitive Therapy Centre, Department of Clinical Psychology, Warneford Hospital, Oxford OX3 7JX, United Kingdom, Phone: (44) 1865 223986; Web: http://www.octc.co.uk

Recommended Reading

Barlow DH, Cerney JA: Psychological Treatment of Panic. New York, Guilford, 1988

Basco MR, Rush AJ: Cognitive-Behavioral Therapy for Bipolar Disorder, 2nd Edition. New York, Guilford, 2005

Beck AT: Love Is Never Enough: How Couples Can Overcome Misunderstandings, Resolve Conflicts, and Solve Relationship Problems Through Cognitive Therapy. New York, Harper & Row, 1988

Beck AT, Freeman A: Cognitive Therapy of Personality Disorders. New York, Guilford, 1990

Beck AT, Rush AJ, Shaw BF, et al: Cognitive Therapy of Depression. New York, Guilford, 1979

Beck AT, Emery GD, Greenberg RL: Anxiety Disorders and Phobias: A Cognitive Perspective. New York, Basic Books, 1985

Beck JS: Cognitive Therapy: Basics and Beyond. New York, Guilford, 1995

Clark DA, Beck AT, Alford BA: Scientific Foundations of Cognitive Theory and Therapy of Depression. New York, Wiley, 1999

Frankl VE: Man's Search for Meaning: An Introduction to Logotherapy, 4th Edition. Boston, Beacon Press, 1992

Freeman A, Simon KM, Beutler LE, et al (eds): Comprehensive Handbook of Cognitive Therapy. New York, Plenum, 1989

Guidano VF, Liotti G: Cognitive Processes and Emotional Disorders: A Structural Approach to Psychotherapy. New York, Guilford, 1983

Kingdon DG, Turkington D: Cognitive Therapy of Schizophrenia. New York, Guilford, 2005

Leahy RL (ed): Contemporary Cognitive Therapy: Theory, Research, and Practice. New York, Guilford, 2004

Linehan MM: Cognitive-Behavioral Treatment of Borderline Personality Disorder. New York, Guilford, 1993

Mahoney MJ, Freeman A (eds): Cognition and Psychotherapy. New York, Plenum, 1985

McCullough JP Jr: Skills Training Manual for Diagnosing and Treating Chronic Depression: Cognitive Behavioral Analysis System of Psychotherapy. New York, Guilford, 2001

Meichenbaum DB: Cognitive-Behavior Modification: An Integrative Approach. New York, Plenum, 1977

Salkovskis PM (ed): Frontiers of Cognitive Therapy. New York, Guilford, 1996

Turk DC, Meichenbaum D, Genest M: Pain and Behavioral Medicine: A Cognitive-Behavioral Perspective. New York, Guilford, 1983

Wright JH (ed): Cognitive-Behavior Therapy (Review of Psychiatry Series, Vol 23; Oldham JM, Riba MB, series eds). Washington DC, American Psychiatric Publishing, 2004

Wright JH, Thase ME, Beck AT, et al (eds): Cognitive Therapy With Inpatients: Developing a Cognitive Milieu. New York, Guilford, 1993

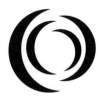

Appendix 3

DVD Guide

Learning Cognitive-Behavior Therapy: An Illustrated Guide

Instructions: Place the DVD in a DVD player or a computer with a DVD drive. A title page will be displayed. Select Menu to view the Menu screens, or wait a few seconds until the Menu screens automatically appear. Select individual videos to view as desired. If you are viewing the DVD on a personal computer, you can click on the right mouse button to display control options such as Menu, Pause, and Play.

Please see the next page for system requirements for DVD playback on a computer (no system requirements are necessary for a DVD player).

System Requirements for DVD Playback on a Computer

Windows XP

Windows Media Player for Windows XP fully supports DVD playback as long as a compatible DVD decoder is installed. Most users with computers that have DVD drives have DVD decoders preinstalled by their hardware manufacturers.

When you insert a DVD movie into your DVD drive for the first time, you'll be prompted to play the DVD movie. If you get an error message when trying to play the DVD with Windows Media Player, you need a DVD decoder. If you bought a PC equipped with a DVD drive, check with the computer manufacturer. The manufacturer may have updated Windows XP DVD decoder drivers available, often for free.

For more information on installing a DVD decoder, visit Microsoft's support website at http://support.microsoft.com, and view article 306331. The article can be found by entering "306331" in the "Search the Knowledge Base" box.

The minimum system requirements for Windows Media Player 10 are as follows:

- Microsoft Windows XP Home Edition, Windows XP Professional, Windows XP Media Center Edition, or Windows XP Tablet PC Edition
- 233 megahertz (MHz) processor or higher, such as an Intel Pentium II or Advanced Micro Devices (AMD) processor
- 64 megabytes (MB) RAM
- 100 MB free hard disk space
- DVD drive with compatible DVD decoder software.
- 28.8 kilobits per second (Kbps) modem
- 16-bit sound card
- Super VGA (800 x 600) monitor resolution
- Video card with 64 MB of RAM (video RAM or VRAM) and DirectX generation
- Speakers or headphones
- Microsoft Internet Explorer 6 or Netscape 7.1

Mac OSX

The following Macintosh models support DVD drives and can play DVD-video discs: Power Mac G5, eMac, PowerBook G4, iBook, iMac, and Mac mini computers. For the latest version of the DVD playback software, visit the following website: http://www.apple.com/macosx/features/dvdplayer.

Video Illustration Number	Video Illustration Title	Time (minutes)
1	Assessing Symptoms of Anxiety: Dr. Wright and Gina	8:40
2	Modifying Automatic Thoughts: Dr. Wright and Gina	10:00
3	Agenda Setting: Dr. Spurgeon and Rose	7:44
4	Psychoeducation on the CBT Model: Dr. Spurgeon and Rose	5:43
5	Psychoeducation on Automatic Thoughts: Dr. Thase and Ed	7:15
6	A Mood Shift: Dr. Fitzgerald and Kris	3:08
7	Guided Discovery: Dr. Fitzgerald and Kris	3:27
8	Imagery: Dr. Fitzgerald and Kris	4:16
9	Generating Rational Alternatives: Dr. Fitzgerald and Kris	6:18
10	Examining the Evidence: Dr. Fitzgerald and Kris	10:15
11	Cognitive Rehearsal: Dr. Fitzgerald and Kris	7:08
12	Activity Scheduling: Dr. Thase and Ed	10:30
13	Graded Task Assignment: Dr. Thase and Ed	7:50
14	Breathing Retraining: Dr. Wright and Gina	7:15
15	Exposure Therapy—Constructing a Hierarchy: Dr. Wright and Gina	10:15
16	In Vivo Exposure Therapy: Dr. Wright and Gina	5:40
17	The Downward Arrow Technique: Dr. Thase and Ed	3:15
18	Examining the Evidence for Schemas: Dr. Thase and Ed	11:00
19	Rehearsing a Modified Schema: Dr. Thase and Ed	7:00
Total Time		136:39

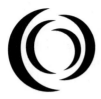

Index

Page numbers printed in **boldface** type refer to tables or figures.